I0791593

Intermittent Fasting
For Health

Lose Weight, Live Long & Unlock Your Body's Potential With Fasting

Taylor Travell

Table of Contents

TABLE OF CONTENTS..7

INTRODUCTION: INTERMITTENT FASTING FOR HEALTH...........1

CHAPTER 1: AN INTRODUCTION TO INTERMITTENT FASTING .6

Fasting is Rooted in Our History 11
Fasting in the Modern World 15

CHAPTER 2: THE INCREDIBLE BENEFITS OF INTERMITTENT FASTING...22

Helps You Lose Weight 23
Optimize Hormone Levels 25
Reduces Inflammation 27
Decreases Oxidative Stress 29
Improves the Biomarkers of Disease......................................30
Reduces the Risk of Developing Various Diseases and Illnesses 31
Improves Insulin Levels and Functions...................................33
Reduce Bad LDL Cholesterol and Blood Triglyceride Levels 35
May Prevent Cancer 36
Facilitates Cellular Repair Processes 38
Modifies the Function and Expression of Certain Genes..........40
Increases the Brain Hormone BDNF 41
Preserves Learning and Memory Functioning.........................42
Reduces Fat in the Liver 44
Increases Endurance, Motor Coordination, and Improves Sleep 45

CHAPTER 3: THE FUNDAMENTALS OF INTERMITTENT FASTING 48

Intermittent Fasting: A Definition...50
Fed State 53

Fasted State...55
The Stages of Intermittent Fasting...........................59

CHAPTER 4: DIFFERENT TYPES OF EATING PATTERNS OF INTERMITTENT FASTING 67

Time-Restricted Fasting Method (16/8 or 14/10)...................69
24-Hour Fasting Method.......................................73
5:2 Fasting Method 76
Warrior Fasting Method 77
Alternate-Day Fasting Method 79
Short-Term vs. Long-Term Fasting Periods 81

CHAPTER 5: MAKING INTERMITTENT FASTING PART OF YOUR LIFESTYLE 88

The Simplicity of IF 90
Establishing IF as Part of Your Lifestyle 91
Where to Start 97
Implementing a Program 103
Addressing the Urge to Eat..................................112
The Importance of Self-Compassion on IF.....................118

CHAPTER 6: THE RISKS, SIDE EFFECTS, AND PRECAUTIONS OF INTERMITTENT FASTING...125

Precautions: What You Need to Know Before Starting IF 127
Typical Side-Effects of IF 137
Safety Tips for Following IF 144

CONCLUSION: INTERMITTENT FASTING AND YOU 148

REFERENCES:...151

Introduction: Intermittent Fasting For Health

"Everyone can perform magic, everyone can reach his goals, if he is able to think, if he is able to wait, if he is able to fast."

— Hermann Hesse, Siddhartha

Have you ever tried going on a diet before?

These days, there are so many different kinds of diets emerging that it can be extremely difficult to choose which one to follow. Having been a health enthusiast for some time now, I had already tried a couple of diets. For a while, I jumped from one diet to another until I found Intermittent Fasting, a diet—more accurately, an eating pattern—that I found to be easy, convenient, and extremely beneficial. To this day, I am still on IF and I couldn't be happier about it. If you're reading this book, then it means that you have some interest in intermittent fasting, so let me tell you more about it.

I know exactly how frustrating it can be to try out different diets without finding success in terms of health and fitness goals. As with any other diet, intermittent fasting isn't for everyone. But I'm sure that you have heard about it by now because it's currently a huge trend. By reading this book, you will learn all the basic information you need to know about intermittent fasting. I have personally experienced the benefits of this diet such as weight loss, balanced hormones, an overall improvement in my health, and more. But before starting, I also researched the potential side effects and risks of the diet to help me determine whether I should start following it or not. To give you the whole picture instead of a biased look at intermittent fasting where only the positives are shown, I will also share these potential side effects and risks with you. In other words, you will learn everything you need to know for you to make a solid decision on whether or not intermittent fasting is your next big lifestyle change.

Of course, since I am an avid follower of intermittent fasting, I will also provide you with lots and lots of tips and strategies to start and stick with this eating pattern. For sure, your intermittent fasting journey will be a lot smoother and easier than mine as I didn't have a self-help book such as this one. I will share my experiences with you along with practical pointers to help you out. With all of the wonderful things I offer you, the next question on your mind may be—who exactly am I and what makes me qualified to share this information?

Well, apart from being a huge fan of intermittent fasting, I do have more to offer. Before we proceed, let me tell you more about myself...

My name is Taylor Travell, 45-years-young (or at least, people tell me I look young) and I work as a dietitian. Ever since I could remember, I was always focused on my health and well-being. Growing up, my whole family was the same way so, naturally, after graduating from high school, I studied nutrition science. A few years later, I got my degree and became a life and fitness coach. As I was studying nutrition science, I became interested in the correlation between the eating behaviors of human beings (both past and present) and how our ancient ancestors used to hunt for food. My research led me to discover the fact that people who lived in the stone age were much healthier, more vital, and had higher energy levels than the average modern man. This was a very interesting discovery that made me delve deeper. Finally, my research proved that the main reason for this health difference originates from the phenomena of forced fasting. I'll explain this more to you later on.

Back then, I was fascinated with the concept of fasting but I didn't think it was for me. So that's when I tried different diets to find which one would make me feel happier and healthier. Also, since eating is an important part of my life (of all our lives, actually), I wanted it to be a positive experience. I didn't want to constantly feel guilty from restricting myself too much. Too often do we hear stories about people failing their diets because they made them feel bad about themselves. I didn't want to end up like that, so I made it my mission to find a diet I was happy to follow.

After all my failed attempts, I circled back to fasting. Intermittent fasting became a trend and I decided to learn everything I could about it. Since nutrition is my passion, I literally read hundreds of resources about it. Don't worry, I won't bore you with too much technical information in this book. As I have said, I only want to share the fundamentals and the most practical strategies that can help you start your own intermittent fasting journey if you choose to by the end of this book. After learning about intermittent fasting and making it part of my lifestyle, I wanted to make my own knowledge and experiences accessible to a wider audience.

Now, I live in London with my husband (who has also started on IF) and two kids. I am happy to say that in terms of diet and health, intermittent fasting was one of the best decisions I've made in my life. I don't stress about the food I eat, I don't have food cravings or obsessions, and I feel free. If you want to experience the same benefits as I have or even more, the best thing you can do is learn. This book is the perfect tool for you and if you choose to continue, then I will be here for you to take this journey with you. With that being said... it's time to start learning!

Chapter 1:

An Introduction to

Intermittent Fasting

For a lot of people, simply hearing the term "fasting" makes them intimidated. But the fact is, fasting is a well-established practice that has been in existence throughout our history. It has been used in different ways and for different purposes, even for therapeutic applications. Today, fasting boasts millions of practitioners and it's also well-received in different kinds of communities. Simply put, fasting is a process wherein you alternate between cycles of eating and not eating (fasting). Several studies and anecdotal reports have shown that fasting can improve your overall health, help you lose weight, protect you against diseases, and even make you live longer. One such study has shown that fasting benefits the cerebrovascular and cardiovascular systems (Mattson & Wan, 2005). Other similar studies have shown promising results, too.

Intermittent fasting isn't really considered a diet, it's more of an eating pattern. This means that the main focus isn't about what you eat, but when you should be eating. With the growing popularity of intermittent fasting, there are several ways to follow it which I will share with you in the next chapters. While the term "intermittent fasting" is new to a lot of people, the basic concept behind it has been around since ancient times. Back then, fasting was mostly done because they had no choice. Over time, people started doing it for a specific purpose.

Because of how popular intermittent fasting (or IF for short) has become, more and more health experts and researchers have started conducting studies about it. Although most of these studies have been done on animals, most of them have shown how safe and effective IF is. Here are some examples of these studies and the promising results they have shown:

- In one study, the researchers discovered that IF causes a good kind of stress on the body (Longo & Mattson, 2014). This stress causes the body's immune system to respond in such a way that it starts repairing cells and it produces a number of positive metabolic changes such as weight loss, reduction in LDL cholesterol, and more.

- Physiologically speaking, fasting can help improve the body's tolerance to different kinds of metabolic stresses (Redman & Ravusinn, 2010). This, in turn, may increase lifespan.
- Compared to other diets, intermittent fasting seems to be very effective in terms of weight loss (Ganesan, Habboush & Sultan, 2018). Although for different study designs, the researchers made use of different IF methods which, in turn, resulted in differed results as well. This shows that the weight loss benefit of intermittent fasting may depend on individuals and on the type of diet followed.

Intermittent fasting may seem intimidating and difficult to follow, but it doesn't have to be. The great thing about this eating pattern is that it's not strict or restrictive like other diets. There are different types of IF eating patterns and you can choose the one which suits your lifestyle the most. After learning about these different methods of following IF, I tried about 2 or 3 methods first before I found the one I felt most comfortable with, and that's the same method I am following now. Another great thing about intermittent fasting is that it has a natural advantage over other diets. Aside from helping you lose weight and maintain a healthy weight long-term, here are some benefits you can expect to experience by following this eating pattern:

- **It promotes blood sugar regulation**

  If you have problems with blood sugar control, intermittent fasting may be the perfect diet for you. Fasting helps improve blood sugar regulation which, in turn, helps reduce your risk of developing diabetes. Fasting helps keep your blood sugar levels steady to prevent crashes and spikes. But for this benefit, it may differ between men and women.

- **It promotes the health of your heart**

  One of the biggest killers in the world right now is heart disease, and this is hugely affected by our diet. Fortunately, intermittent fasting can help improve the risk factors of heart disease like inflammatory markers, blood pressure, LDL cholesterol, and more.

- **It helps slow down the process of aging**

Many benefits of intermittent fasting are similar to the positive effects and benefits of a low-calorie diet. This is why IF can help slow down the aging process. Aside from helping with the prevention and treatment of diseases, fasting stimulates adaptive stress responses in the cells which, in turn, enhances your body's ability to combat diseases and cope with stress. These effects are what mainly provide anti-aging benefits. That's probably why I get a lot of compliments for looking younger than I actually am!

- **It may help you live a longer life**

This is one of the more exciting benefits of intermittent fasting. In several studies conducted on animals, the results have shown that IF extends the lifespan of animals in the same way as continuously following a low-calorie diet. But the difference is, you won't have to limit yourself in terms of the types of food you have to eat. This is why intermittent fasting is a lot easier to stick with compared to other diets.

As with any other diet, intermittent fasting works incredibly well with some people, but not for everyone. Fortunately, intermittent fasting worked well for me and I am now very happy and comfortable with this eating pattern. Hopefully, if you decide to start IF too, it gives you all of these benefits and more!

Fasting is Rooted in Our History

As I have already mentioned, fasting has been around since ancient times. While people in the past had fasted out of necessity, over the years, people have started seeing the benefits of deliberate fasting. Because of this, fasting has changed, evolved, and has now become one of the most popular health and fitness trends all over the world.

The fact is, fasting is deeply rooted in our history. As one of the most ancient practices, even Hippocrates of Cos prescribed it, especially when suffering from an illness. According to Hippocrates, eating while you are sick is feeding your illness. Plutarch, another famous person from ancient Greece, also shared these sentiments. For him, it was better to fast when sick instead of taking medicine to treat the sickness. Even Plato and Aristotle were strong supporters of this ancient tradition. When it comes to famous advocates of fasting, the list goes on.

In the past, our ancient ancestors procured their food by fishing, hunting, or gathering. These ancestral hunter-gatherers would fast while foraging until they either caught, killed, or found their food. Unlike today, people in the past didn't have the luxury of having breakfast, lunch, dinner or even snacks ready at specific times of the day. Since food wasn't readily available, our ancestors ate opportunistically as long as they could get their hands on any kind of food. Also, unlike today, most humans only ate 1 to 2 meals a day...imagine that! Although they may have wanted to eat more frequently, food was scarce—and so they had no choice but to fast.

As the years went by and food became more abundant, fasting remained to be a part of our lives. This time, fasting became a very significant part of spiritual and religious practices. In fact, these purposes of fasting have already been a part of our customs as human beings since prehistory. We know this because it is mentioned in most of the spiritual books of different religions.

Traditionally, those who fast for religious or spiritual purposes do so for purification or to atone for their sins. For most religions, there are certain seasons or days when their believers are supposed to fast, and again, this is done for specific purposes. Here are some examples of religions that promote fasting as part of their beliefs:

- **Baha'i**

  For Baha'is, their fasting season occurs during "Ala." This is the 19th month of their Baha'i year and it falls on the 2nd of March to the 20th of March.

- **Buddhist**

  All of the main Buddhist sects practice periods of fasting. Usually, these are done on holidays or during full-moon days.

- **Catholic**

  Devout Catholics fast during the Lenten season, specifically on Ash Wednesday and on Good Friday. Aside from this, they also abstain from eating meat on all Fridays of the season.

- **Hinduism**

Hindus have a lot of fasting days that usually occur on new moon days. They also fast during festivals like Puja, Shivaratri, Saraswati, and so on.

- **Judaism**

The Day of Atonement which is also known as "Yom Kippur" is the most well-known day of fasting for the Jewish people. Their calendar has other days of fasting too, 6 more to be exact.

Another popular reason for fasting is for treatment or healing. This is known as therapeutic fasting and it's meant to either prevent or treat illnesses. Fasting under medical supervision gained popularity back in the 19th century in the US as part of the "Natural Hygiene Movement." In fact, in the year 1928, Dr. Herbert Shelton opened a Health School in Texas which has helped thousands of patients become healthier through water fasting. In the UK, fasting became part of an approach known as "Nature Cure" that emphasized the importance of positive thinking, fresh air, sunshine, exercise, and a healthy diet.

Because people had seen and experienced all the benefits of fasting time and again through the years, it endured. Now, the newest trend in fasting is intermittent fasting which, in itself, comes with a lot of variations. Intermittent fasting isn't a new thing—it's another evolution of the ancient practice that has been a part of our lives as human beings from the very beginning.

Fasting in the Modern World

If you plan to join me and the countless others who are following the intermittent fasting trend, you now know that this practice has been around since time immemorial. In our modern-day society, a lot of people consider it "fashionable" to fast for their health. This is why intermittent fasting has surged in popularity. When celebrities and influencers started joining the trend, more and more people wanted in on it, too. Today, millions of people fast, including those following IF.

Among all the reasons for fasting, one of the most important and enduring is for religion. When it comes to religion, fasting involves either partially or completely abstaining from the consumption of food for a specific number of days. It is one of the most ancient practices that exists in most of the world's religions. Recently, various studies have shown that fasting is beneficial for health. When practiced correctly and with caution, it may bring about heightened states of sensibility and consciousness. Also, most religions recommend their adherents to accompany their fasting with prayers.

Even now, some people believe that fasting is one way to wake up the spiritual and physical parts of the body to promote healing. Even fasting for a single day can provide you with a lot of benefits. Fasting can help "reset" your body and your psyche. Now, more people who work in the fields of healing claim that medical procedures can work more efficiently when the mental, spiritual, physical, and emotional aspects of a person are aligned—and fasting helps promote this alignment.

When it comes to fasting in religion, Islam is one of the leaders in its reformation. This religion made fasting easier, more effective, and more natural. In the past, fasting symbolized mourning, sadness, an atonement for their sins, and even as a reminder of past disasters. Then the Muslims radicalized this concept and transformed it into a more enlightened concept of positivity and self-purification. Muslims fast for a whole month accompanied by worship and welcoming the new year with happiness and energy.

To this day, the governing laws of fasting in Islam are universal and fair. Unlike other religions, Islam permits all adults to fast irrespective of their social status or class. In particular, this religion has one tradition known as "sehri" which is the meal eaten before the beginning of the fast. This is an excellent example of how Islam has made the practice easy for their people to follow. Here, people who are fasting can eat until just a couple of minutes before they say their morning prayer. Then when the sun has set, they can break the fast and celebrate. Muslims are also allowed to rest and sleep throughout the day while they are fasting. But they don't have to stop working or close their businesses while fasting. Basically, it just means that they can continue with their daily lives and routines with the only change being that they won't take breaks to eat meals. Furthermore, when they break their fast by mistake, they are forgiven for it, not punished.

Of course, Islam isn't the only religion in this modern time where their adherents practice fasting. I just stated this example to show you that fasting doesn't have to be a difficult or negative thing. For Muslims, this is part of their tradition and they have come to accept it and even look forward to it because of its significance in their belief system. In the same way, you can make the conscious choice to make intermittent fasting part of your life. You don't have to rush the process nor should you force yourself into it. One thing you can count on when you decide to follow intermittent fasting is that you aren't alone.

The first time intermittent fasting went mainstream was back in 2012. Michael Mosley, a doctor and journalist based in the UK, published a book about it. For most people, weight loss is the most common benefit they are looking to get from IF. But two students from Yale who practiced IF also shared that fasting made them less obsessed with food. By following the eating pattern, they reduced their cravings which, in turn, allowed them to focus on other things.

Intermittent fasting refers to a number of approaches wherein you would abstain from food short-term to improve your health. I would like to emphasize the fact that this is "short-term" because IF doesn't involve fasting for long periods of time.

There are some notable works out there written earlier than this one that talk about intermittent fasting. For one, Dr. Michael Mosley wrote a book entitled *Eat Fast, Live Longer and The Fast Diet* in 2012 and it focused mainly on the 5:2 IF method (we'll go through these different methods later). Here, Mosley emphasized that IF is a simple eating pattern that doesn't involve complicated rules. It's a user-friendly, flexible, and comprehensible diet that allows you to eat the foods you love. This makes it more sustainable in the long-run.

Another noteworthy book was written by Dr. Jason Fung in 2016 entitled *The Obesity Code*. Here, Fung suggested that the underlying cause of obesity isn't an excess of calories. While cutting down on caloric intake may cause one to lose weight, this isn't a long-term solution. According to Fung, the real issue behind this condition is an imbalance of hormones in the body caused by years of bad eating habits. Fortunately, bringing hormonal balance to the body is one of the benefits of intermittent fasting, too.

Because of how hugely popular intermittent fasting is right now, we have seen an increase in interest from the scientific and medical community. This is why there are a lot of recent studies and research done about it. IF is also widely popular in the health and fitness community along with those interested in life-hacking strategies. This is probably why you chose to purchase this book in the first place—to learn more about it so you can determine whether it's right for you or not. One thing I can say to you about intermittent fasting right now is that it can make things a lot easier for you diet-wise while improving your overall health.

Chapter 2:

The Incredible Benefits of Intermittent Fasting

Even before reading this book, you have probably heard about intermittent fasting already. By now, after learning the rich history of fasting, you are getting a clearer picture of this eating pattern and why it is so enduring. Intermittent fasting won't just allow you to save time and money, but it will also provide you with a host of health benefits without having to change your life drastically or sacrifice the foods you love. Probably the biggest issue you will encounter here (at least as per experience) is the adjustment of not eating as frequently as you did in the past. But this isn't an issue you will experience for a long time. The more you stick with this diet, the faster you will be able to adapt to this new way of eating.

Before starting a new diet, you want to learn why you should do so. I don't blame you. I myself had researched the benefits of intermittent fasting before I started following it. Because of my research, I have learned all about these benefits and in this chapter, I will share the most important ones with you. Since my aim here is to give you a realistic look at intermittent fasting, I will inform you which of these benefits have already been proven and which are highly possible but may require more studies to prove definitively. Hopefully, this will help you out in terms of making a decision on whether you want to start following the diet or not. Here are the benefits of this worldwide trend:

Helps You Lose Weight

A lot of people who start following intermittent fasting want to lose weight. When you think about it, this makes a lot of sense. Since you will be eating fewer meals throughout the day, you will definitely lose weight. That is, unless you try to compensate by overeating during your feasting window. This is a big no-no that you should try to avoid as much as possible. Aside from naturally reducing your caloric intake, IF also improves the functions of your hormones to promote weight loss.

Intermittent fasting promotes changes in the body that help you shed weight a lot faster. In one study, the researchers discovered that fasting can increase your metabolic rate by as much as 14%, thus helping your body burn more calories (Zauner, et. al., 2000). It's also important to note that intermittent fasting helps you lose belly fat, the harmful type of fat located in your abdominal cavity. Combine this improved ability to burn more calories with your consistent reduction of caloric intake to get a very powerful aid for weight loss. Now combine this winning combination with regular exercise and a healthy, balanced diet and you will see this benefit in no time!

One interesting fact that I had stumbled upon while reading about the weight loss benefit of IF is that when you take long breaks from food, this doesn't just speed up metabolism. It also causes the conversion of body fat into brown fat, a healthier type of fat that aids in the fat-burning process. The more brown fat you have in your body, the more it becomes a fat-burning machine. Soon, you may notice your fat stores being burned away instead of getting accumulated in the different parts of your body. This is one of the most common and most celebrated benefits of intermittent fasting and it's one that I have personally experienced.

Optimize Hormone Levels

Did you know that hormonal imbalances can cause a lot of issues with your health? Even a small imbalance in your hormones can cause a huge impact. Since IF can help optimize your hormone levels, this is one of the best benefits the eating pattern has to offer. While there is a lot of anecdotal evidence about this benefit, there is a need for further research to solidify this claim. Most IF enthusiasts see it as a "magic bullet" to improve health, but as with any other diet, proof from studies and research can help build its credibility, especially for those who are still on the fence when it comes to deciding whether they want to join the trend.

One particular study I found that had a direct relation to this benefit showed that intermittent fasting helped improve hormone levels (Wei, et. al. 2017). The researchers saw this through the reduction of the risk factors and markers of disease and aging. Many of the other studies focused on the impact of intermittent fasting on hormones have been conducted on animals or on small groups of people at the peak of their health. But when it comes to anecdotal reports, you will find a lot of these out there. Here are some ways intermittent fasting can help with your hormones:

- An increase in the production of the growth hormone to help repair muscle mass and burn body fat.
- A reduction in the release of ghrelin and leptin, the hunger hormones. This is why you experience a reduction in food cravings after some time.
- For women, an improvement in progesterone and estrogen levels, the female sex hormones.
- A decrease in cortisol levels and an increase in melatonin levels. This helps lower your stress while improving your sleep.
- An improvement in thyroid hormone levels. This is very important as these hormones have an effect on all of your body's cells.

These are just some examples of how intermittent fasting can be beneficial to your hormones. To enhance these benefits, you may want to choose whole and unprocessed foods instead of opting for unhealthy food options all the time.

Reduces Inflammation

This is another significant benefit since inflammation is a key factor in the development of chronic diseases. Several studies have shown that intermittent fasting can combat inflammation. Although acute inflammation is normal and it can help protect your body against diseases and infections, chronic inflammation can have severe and detrimental consequences on your health.

One of the more recent studies about IF concluded that it can really help reduce inflammation in the body (Jordan, et. al., 2019). According to this study, this reduction occurred along with the reduction of a type of cell in the body known as "monocytes." These cells cause inflammation but through intermittent fasting, the number of these cells in the blood can lower significantly. Also, researchers discovered that the monocytes in the blood were not as inflammatory as in those who didn't follow the diet. However, this was another study conducted on mice.

There are other studies that have shown that skipping meals helps lower inflammation to promote better health. Some of these studies have focused specifically on intermittent fasting and these have shown that following the diet for at least a month can already decrease inflammatory marker levels dramatically. Imagine how this diet will improve your life if you follow it long-term? One important thing to note here is that if you want to enjoy this benefit, you should avoid overeating as much as you can. This is especially true at the beginning of your diet. In fact, this is one piece of advice that will help you with all the other benefits. After all, even if you stick with your fasting schedule but you constantly binge and eat unhealthy foods when it's time for you to eat, don't expect your health to improve. As with any other type of diet, the key here is moderation and making healthier choices.

Decreases Oxidative Stress

Apart from inflammation, oxidative stress is another important factor that contributes to the development of various diseases. In fact, this is one of the things that hastens the aging process and makes you more vulnerable to chronic diseases. Throughout our lives, the cells of our body may encounter damage. One way this happens is through oxidative stress. Oxidative stress occurs when there is an abundance of free radicals in your body. These are unstable molecules carrying electrons that are highly reactive. When these free radicals come in contact with other molecules, this may cause a very quick chain reaction that causes the formation of more free radicals. When this happens, the connections between your body's atoms and cells are damaged or even broken.

Intermittent fasting seems to be very helpful in helping your cells combat oxidative stress. However, researchers and health experts aren't clear on how this happens exactly. Some believe that fasting causes the body's cells to activate survival processes to eliminate unhealthy or damaged cells (or cell parts) and replace these with healthy ones. Over time, this reduces the production of free radicals in the body. In other words, it's like a chain reaction but in reverse.

One study focused on the benefits of intermittent fasting in terms of combating oxidative stress had shown that fasting can, in fact, reduce the levels of oxidative stress in the body (Nurmasitoh, et. al., 2018). This, in turn, helps decrease the risk of developing degenerative and chronic diseases. In another study, this time focused on fasting done by Muslims during Ramadan, researchers came to the conclusion that this fasting stimulates positive metabolic changes in the body (Farris, et. al., 2012). This helps the body adapt to the alteration of feeding patterns done during this holy fasting month. Although fasting for a month is different from making the choice to fast long-term, you may experience this benefit, too.

Improves the Biomarkers of Disease

One of the most significant indicators of your overall well-being and health is how efficient your biological processes are. When everything works well, this means that your body operates efficiently and all your hormones and chemicals are balanced. If not, this is when you may experience physical symptoms or medical conditions. Intermittent fasting can help improve your metabolic efficiency. This happens when your glucose supply gets depleted so your body starts metabolizing your fat stores. IF also has a positive effect on the regulation of important hormones and chemicals in your body.

In one study, researchers discovered that intermittent fasting helps improve metabolic health (Patterson, et. al., 2015). Naturally, this benefit also comes with the improvement of the various risk factors or biomarkers of diseases. As with most of the other benefits here, a lot of studies conducted about intermittent fasting have focused on animals. The important thing is that these studies have indicated that this benefit is, in fact, highly probable. This is especially true if you opt for healthier food options whenever it's time for you to eat. I cannot stress the importance of your food options enough. Just because you're following IF, that doesn't mean that you should gorge on processed or junk foods. If you want to experience all the good stuff, gradually change your eating habits along with your eating patterns. Trust me, it will all be worth the effort.

Reduces the Risk of Developing Various Diseases and Illnesses

You have probably experienced falling ill at least once in your life. Do you remember the time when you felt really sick? During that time, you may have noticed that your appetite wasn't as robust as it normally was. Even when other animals get sick, they have a tendency to stop eating (or fast) while they are recovering. And have you noticed that despite not eating, you get better? This is because periods of fasting can help you stay healthy.

Do you know why?

Several studies have shown that intermittent fasting can help lower blood pressure and bad cholesterol levels, promote fat- and glucose-burning faster, increase insulin sensitivity, and more. All of these help reduce the risk of developing various diseases and illnesses like diabetes, heart disease, multiple sclerosis, and more. Apart from these benefits, intermittent fasting can also give your immune system a boost, thus keeping you protected from all kinds of potential illnesses.

As long as you follow intermittent fasting properly (it's easy, don't worry), it can help reduce your chances of developing long-term health problems. Even if you're suffering from medical conditions right now, you can improve your health through intermittent fasting. One word of caution though—if you have any kind of medical condition, consult with your doctor first before following any diet, even intermittent fasting. Healthy as this diet is, you should always put your own safety first. Your doctor can even help you decide which method of IF to choose.

Improves Insulin Levels and Functions

These days, type 2 diabetes has become a very common problem and one of the main features of this condition is high levels of blood sugar. Interestingly enough, intermittent fasting can help improve your insulin resistance by lowering the levels of your blood sugar. Some studies conducted on human beings regarding intermittent fasting have shown that following this eating pattern can help lower the levels of blood sugar by as much as 6% while the levels of fasting insulin have gone down by as much as 31%.

According to the Centers for Disease Control and Prevention in the US, more than 84 million people in the country already suffer from a condition called pre-diabetes. If left unchecked and untreated, this condition may lead to type 2 diabetes in a matter of 5 years. One way to prevent this from happening is by losing weight, especially for overweight or obese individuals. By losing weight, your body becomes more sensitive to insulin. As we have already discussed, one of the most common benefits of intermittent fasting is weight loss...but that's not all.

Each time you eat, your insulin is released into your bloodstream to give energy to your cells. But if you have pre-diabetes, this makes you insulin-resistant. This means that your blood levels tend to remain elevated all the time. Through intermittent fasting, you reduce your body's need to produce insulin all the time. If you suffer from pre-diabetes, you already have diabetes or you have a family history of this condition, intermittent fasting can be very helpful to you. In one particular study, researchers discovered that intermittent fasting can help restore the secretion of insulin (Cheng et. al., 2017). This may also help promote the production of new beta cells in the pancreas that produce insulin. While there is a need for further research on this benefit, earlier studies conducted on cell samples of human beings have shown similar promising results. Diabetes is a lifelong condition that can be very difficult. So anything that can help improve the management of this condition can also improve the quality of your life.

Reduce Bad LDL Cholesterol and Blood Triglyceride Levels

High LDL cholesterol and blood triglyceride levels are risk factors for heart disease. According to the Centers for Disease Control and Prevention, more than 600,000 people in the US die of heart disease each year. To reduce this risk, you can quit smoking, limit your alcohol intake, exercise regularly, and follow a healthier diet—like intermittent fasting. Research has shown that restricting calories each day doesn't just help improve insulin resistance and glycemic control, but it also helps improve your cardiovascular risk.

Since intermittent fasting can help you lose weight, this also comes with cardiovascular benefits. This is actually why I listed weight loss as the first benefit of IF, because it has a positive effect on all the other benefits. As you lose weight, you may also see an improvement in the triglyceride and LDL cholesterol concentrations in your body. This is a different pattern of eating that doesn't restrict you too much or make you feel like you're "on a diet."

In one particular review, researchers found out that intermittent fasting can, in fact, result in the reduction of triglyceride, cholesterol, heart rate, and blood pressure levels (Mattson, Longo & Harvie, 2017). This time, the study came up with this conclusion for animals and for human beings. Other similar studies conducted on humans and animals have revealed positive results as well. Because of all these studies and the many anecdotal reports, intermittent fasting is now associated with a lower risk of developing heart disease, thanks to these level reductions.

May Prevent Cancer

Cancer is probably one of the scariest and most terrible diseases in existence and it's characterized by an uncontrollable growth of (cancer) cells. Although there is still a need for further research to prove this benefit, several animal studies have shown promising results indicating that intermittent fasting may help prevent the development or spread of cancer. This may be due to the fact that intermittent fasting provides a lot of positive effects on metabolism.

There have been some small studies done on humans about how intermittent fasting can positively affect this disease, too. In one particular study, the researchers focused on the 5:2 method of intermittent fasting (Harvie, et. al., 2016). The results of the study showed that this form can initiate physical changes in the body that may lead to a reduction in the risk of developing cancer, particularly breast cancer. Other studies have shown that intermittent fasting can help prevent tumor formation and growth. Also, some evidence from studies has shown that fasting can help reduce the adverse side effects chemotherapy has on the body. This means that if you already suffer from cancer and you're undergoing chemotherapy, you may want to ask your doctor about starting on IF.

Personally, I have not experienced this benefit since I am lucky enough not to suffer from this disease. However, as I was doing research, this always came up probably because it's another important benefit that can help a lot of people all over the world. Cancer is a disease with no known cure. Once you or one of your loved ones gets it, the experience can be devastating. So if there is anything that can help reduce the risk or improve the condition, I believe that it's worth knowing about. If you are particularly interested in this benefit, you can keep an eye out for further research as these may provide more concrete evidence and results.

Facilitates Cellular Repair Processes

One important effect of intermittent fasting occurs within the cells. This is a process of waste removal known as "autophagy" wherein the cells break down the dysfunctional proteins that accumulated inside them (the cells) over time. After that, the cells then metabolize these proteins. When there is an increase in this process within your body, this provides you with protection against different kinds of diseases.

Autophagy is an important process your body needs to stay healthy. But you should know that as soon as you start eating again, this process comes to a halt. This is because proteins, insulin, and glucose cause the cessation of autophagy. The next time you fast, this gives your body time to continue with the waste removal process, thus keeping your body healthy. You can think of this process as a janitor working in an office building who isn't able to clean when it is fully occupied. But as soon as everyone takes a break or goes home for the day, the janitor can sweep, mop, dust, and polish in peace. This helps keep the building clean and well-maintained.

For this benefit, though, you need to be careful. While fasting can promote your health, depriving your body of nourishing food for long periods of time isn't ideal either. After removing all the waste, your body needs to be nourished to replenish whatever has been lost. Instead of starving yourself to lose weight and experience all the other benefits of fasting, choose to consume healthier foods and beverages whenever it's time for you to eat. That way, your body and all its cells are nourished by the food you eat rather than getting damaged because of harmful free radicals from unhealthy, processed food. If you're fond of these types of food, try to wean yourself off them gradually. That way, you won't feel like you're depriving yourself as you start on IF.

Modifies the Function and Expression of Certain Genes

During fasting, several things start happening in your body. One of these things is the modification of the expression and function of certain genes. This benefit has a very scientific nature to it, but I'll try to explain it to you in a way that's easy to understand. Through IF, you will experience a number of beneficial changes in different molecules and genes related to disease protection and longevity. For one, fasting stimulates your SIRT3 gene to increase the production of protective proteins called sirtuins which are associated with longevity. Basically, this means that modifications that occur in certain genes may help improve your aging process. Of course, there are other benefits as well in terms of genes, but researchers and scientists are still in the process of discovering these.

Increases the Brain Hormone BDNF

With all the benefits intermittent fasting has to offer your body, you might be wondering, "what about my brain?" Well, whatever is beneficial to your body will be beneficial for your brain, too. Intermittent fasting can help improve different metabolic features that are important for the health of the brain such as an improvement in insulin resistance, lowered levels of blood sugar, and more.

A number of studies have also revealed that IF may promote the growth of new brain cells which, in turn, improves the functions of the brain too. Following this eating pattern can even elevate the levels of brain-derived neurotrophic factor or BDNF, a type of brain hormone. Low levels or a deficiency of this brain hormone has been associated with different kinds of brain issues and conditions.

Some research (again, limited to animals) has revealed that IF can have a powerful effect on the health of the brain in terms of structure and function. And since one of the benefits of IF is a reduction of inflammation, it can also help prevent the development of neurodegenerative disorders such as Parkinson's and Alzheimer's. But as with other benefits, more research is needed—especially on humans—to solidify these claims.

Preserves Learning and Memory Functioning

Still related to brain health, intermittent fasting can increase the occurrence of autophagy. I have already explained how autophagy is a process of waste removal and this occurs in the brain cells, too. Because IF initiates this process, you may see an improvement in your memory, learning, and other cognitive functions. Some studies conducted on rats have shown that when they are subjected to fasting, their cells experience minor levels of stress. When this happens, their cells' reaction is to enhance their stress coping abilities. This can help improve the resistance of the brain to neurodegenerative disorders.

While there have been several studies conducted about the benefits of intermittent fasting on the brain, one particular study had focused on how hunger modulates the functions of the brain (Cerqueira, Chausse & Kowaltowski, 2017). According to the results of this study, fasting can either prevent or delay the onset of neurodegenerative diseases. In fact, the researchers even reported that intermittent fasting benefits not just the functions of the brain, but its integrity as well. The fact is, your brain is very sensitive to fasting because it requires a lot of energy as it controls all the actions of the body! This means that when you fast, it's your brain that experiences most of the effects and benefits. And since there are a lot of benefits, this means that IF is really brain-friendly.

I have used the term neurodegenerative disorders and the most famous (and most common) of these is Alzheimer's disease. As with cancer, this is a condition with no cure, therefore, prevention is key. Fortunately, several studies done on animals and some on humans have shown that intermittent fasting can help delay the onset of this disease. Furthermore, pairing IF with other healthy lifestyle changes can help improve the symptoms and make the disease more manageable. The diet can also help protect you from similar diseases like Huntington's disease, Parkinson's disease, and so on.

Reduces Fat in the Liver

Recent studies have shed light on the significance of when we eat (this means our eating patterns or schedules), not just what or how much we eat. These studies have shown that intermittent fasting can reduce the risk of another common type of disease that is caused by high amounts of fat in the liver. Non-alcoholic fatty liver disease is a diet-related condition millions of people suffer from and a lot of them aren't even aware of it. Left unchecked and untreated, this disease can lead to other chronic or metabolic diseases.

Through intermittent fasting, your liver cells become mildly stressed. This, in turn, stimulates the production of GADD45β, which, in turn, adjusts your metabolism to accommodate the low intake of food. This benefit is supported by a study done on rodents (Hatori, et. al., 2012). The benefit here occurs because GADD45β hinders the uptake of fatty acids in the liver to improve your metabolic health.

While intermittent fasting can help prevent the development of non-alcoholic fatty liver disease, those who suffer from it can also enjoy this benefit. By following IF, there is a possibility of reversing the disease by simply making modifications in your eating pattern or schedule. Fasting may also increase gene expression, particularly of the genes that prevent the accumulation of triglycerides in your liver. This is yet another significant benefit of IF that will help you become healthier in the long run.

Increases Endurance, Motor Coordination, and Improves Sleep

At the beginning of your intermittent fasting journey, it's not a good idea to continue with your normal workout regimen, especially if it involves moderate to high-intensity exercises. Since you won't be consuming as much as you did in the past, it's not safe for you to exercise strenuously while fasting. Otherwise, you might end up feeling fatigued. In some cases, you might even experience muscle loss as your body starts breaking down your protein stores for energy—which are your muscles.

Over time, as your body adjusts to your new eating patterns, you will notice that your motor coordination and endurance will start increasing. For this benefit to happen, you have to give your body time. Think about it this way—when you are learning a new skill, you take time to practice so that you can master the skill, right? In the same way, your body needs time to get used to your new eating pattern as well as the prolonged periods of time when you don't eat. When it comes to exercising and working out while following intermittent fasting, you have to be smart about it. Pay close attention to your body so you can determine the best kind of workout to follow and the best time to work out.

As intermittent fasting benefits your overall health and metabolism, it can also help bring balance to your circadian rhythms. And when this happens, your metabolism improves even more. After deciding which schedule or method to follow, stick with it so your body gets used to it. Then, over time, your circadian rhythm catches up and you will be able to sleep better, too. Harmonizing your eating patterns with your circadian rhythm helps improve your weight regulation as well. With all of these great benefits, you'll notice that you're able to fall asleep faster at night and stay asleep throughout the night. Personally, this is one of the benefits I had noticed and it also happens to be one of the benefits I appreciate the most because before I started on IF, I experienced a lot of sleeping difficulties.

Chapter 3

The Fundamentals of

Intermittent Fasting

As you can see, fasting spurs a number of biological responses in your body and these are what cause all of the wonderful benefits. The great thing about intermittent fasting is that the longer you stick with it, the more your body gets used to it. And the more your body gets used to intermittent fasting, the more you will start experiencing the numerous benefits. Some of these benefits even lead to more good things for your health. Now that you have a better idea of how this diet can improve your overall health, you may feel more excited about following it.

Now that I have gotten you more excited about IF, it's time for you to learn more about it. Learning the basics of this unique eating pattern will help you understand it better. Here, I will define what intermittent fasting is in a way that hopefully is simple and easy to understand. When I was trying to learn about IF, I had encountered a lot of technical definitions and those made my head spin. But then, I was also able to read some enlightening resources that explained what IF is all about in the simplest possible way.

As I came to understand what IF really is and was successfully able to apply it to my life, I can confidently share this information, too. Let me explain what IF is all about along with the fed and fasted states and the different stages you will undergo as you begin your own journey. That way, you will have a better idea of what to expect as things unfold.

Intermittent Fasting: A Definition

Let me reiterate this fact once again—intermittent fasting or simply IF is more of a lifestyle or eating pattern instead of a diet. Although I refer to it as a diet once in a while, this just makes it easier for me and the readers. But in reality, IF focuses more on when you will eat instead of what you should eat or how much your portions should be. Simply put, to follow this diet means that you make a conscious choice to skip meals according to the fasting schedule you have set for yourself. Therefore, you would only consume all the calories and nutrients your body needs during a specific timeframe commonly known as the "feasting window." As this window comes to an end, this is when your "fasting window" begins. The time you set for fasting is typically longer to give your body time to provide all of the benefits we discussed in the previous chapter.

It's as simple as that!

After understanding the simplicity of the diet, I went back to the technical explanations and when I read them again, I started to understand them too. No matter how you put it, intermittent fasting is all about changing your usual eating patterns to make them more deliberate. Now that this is clearer for you, the next question you may have on your mind is..."Is it safe?"

Intermittent fasting isn't perfect. Even though fasting as a practice has been around since ancient times, this doesn't mean that it's completely safe and free of risks. Later on, we will be discussing these in more detail. Generally, though, if you follow IF correctly, it can be both safe and beneficial. When I say "follow it correctly," I mean that you choose an IF method that you believe will suit your lifestyle best (after trying out the different methods first), you stick with it as much as you can, and try to clean up your diet too. Also, make sure that you get all the nutrients your body needs to stay healthy within your fasting window. That way, you don't end up becoming deficient in any essential vitamins, minerals, or nutrients.

One word of caution: if you restrict yourself too much, you might start experiencing adverse side effects. For instance, if your main goal for following IF is to lose weight and you do this by eating very little during your feasting window each day. While this will definitely make you lose weight, it will not be in the right way. Severe caloric restriction is a huge no-no in IF or any other type of diet for that matter. When you develop a nutrient deficiency, this may lead to a number of medical problems.

When followed correctly and when you learn how to listen to your body as you are fasting intermittently, this is when you can expect to enjoy all the benefits. IF is very beneficial because your body works in a different way during your fasting and feasting windows. Each time you consume a meal, it takes a couple of hours for your body to process everything. Through this process, your body breaks down your food and turns it into energy for your body to use. This type of energy is readily available, thus your body utilizes it instead of using the fat stores you have in the different parts of your body.

But when you start fasting, your body doesn't have this readily available energy to use. Since it needs energy for the different processes to keep working, your body turns to your fat stores. These are the ones being broken down for fuel and these are the ones your body runs on during your fasting window.

But what does this all mean?

Essentially, intermittent fasting helps your body learn how to utilize the food you eat in a more efficient way. Over time, your body will start learning how to burn your fat stores for fuel whenever you fast. As you follow IF, your body will constantly cycle in and out of two states—the fed state and the fasted state. For you to understand these states better, let's go through them separately.

Fed State

The fed state is also referred to as the "absorptive state" and it occurs after you consume food. Then your body starts digesting the food you ate so that it can absorb all the nutrients. But what you may not know is that even thinking about, smelling, or seeing food can start the process of digestion. Specifically, as soon as your mouth starts watering, this is when digestion begins. Then as you eat and even after you're done, the process continues until all of the nutrients have been transported to the different organs in your body. Usually, the fed state lasts around 4 hours after eating. During this time, your body is already absorbing the nutrients, either utilizing them or converting them to energy for storage. When your body is in the fed state, your glucose levels increase which, in turn, increases insulin secretion, too. The insulin that is released gets attached to the glucose then transports it to your cells for utilization. But it can also get transported to the muscles and liver to be converted then stored for the future.

Throughout the fed state, your insulin levels remain elevated. This stimulates your body to start storing excess calories in your fat cells. Also, while insulin levels are high, your body doesn't burn fat because it has enough energy to use from the food you've just eaten.

Now, try to think about what your body does with your current diet.

Let's say that throughout your day, you eat 3 meals (breakfast, lunch, and dinner) plus snacks in between. Since the fed state lasts even after you have eaten and it doesn't end until your body has used up all the energy from your food, this means that the time this state ends may vary. If you eat a huge meal, your fed state would last a lot longer compared to when you eat a light meal or snack. But if you eat something between your main meals, this means that your body would continue to be in the fed state all throughout the day. Naturally, since there is an excess of calories coming in because of how much and how frequently you eat, your body turns all of this excess into fat.

Even if you follow such a diet, there is still a time when you naturally fast within the day—when you go to sleep. Unless you never sleep, you naturally go into the fasting state each night when you catch some shut-eye. Since you aren't eating while sleeping, the processes within your body start to change. Even without readily available energy stores to rely on, you don't end up starving to death. This is because your body still has energy stored in different places and this is what is used during the fasted state. Naturally, the processes that happen during the fasted state while you sleep are the same processes that happen when you deliberately fast because you're on IF. Let's learn more about this next state and why it's so significant.

Fasted State

Although fasting has been around for ages now, conventional wisdom led a lot of us to believe that when you skip meals to lose weight (or for any other purpose), this is an unsustainable method that will ultimately lead to crash dieting, yo-yo dieting, binge eating, and other unhealthy habits that will prevent you from reaching your health and fitness goals. But when you make IF part of your lifestyle, it can potentially lead to a healthier body and mind. This is because when your body enters the fasted state—an important aspect of IF—a number of things start to occur.

As soon as the fed state comes to an end, the fasted or postabsorptive state begins. This state occurs after all of the food you have eaten has completely undergone digestion, absorption, and storage. Once in a fasted state, your body turns to your glycogen stores to continue operating normally. Because of this, your blood glucose levels go down as your cells start using your energy stores to function. This causes your levels of insulin to go down too. When your blood glucose levels continue to drop, this stimulates the pancreas to produce and secrete glucagon, which is a type of hormone. Once secreted, glucagon is transported to your liver for the purpose of breaking down your glycogen stores into glucose. After this, your liver releases glucose to be used by the different parts of the body for energy. The thing that triggers your body to switch from using food as your energy source to using stores for fuel is the fall of insulin levels.

Let me share an example with you to make this clearer. For instance, let's say you fast for 24 hours straight (there is an IF method wherein you would do this). As your body goes into the fasting state, you still require 2,000 calories for that day to keep your body going. If you have a lot of fat stores, then your body can easily survive the day. Around half a pound of body fat can supply you with the 2,000 calories you need and if you have more than that, then you can continue with this type of IF method. The fasting state is a natural state of the body that occurs when you stop eating either deliberately or not. Then when you start eating again, your body goes back to the fed state.

When it comes to fat, your body either uses it or stores it, but these processes can't occur simultaneously. If you eat a lot of food, your body stores all the excess. This is when you start noticing the different parts of your body getting bigger. But when food is scarce and your body feels deprived, this is when your body becomes a fat-burning machine. For this process, the key regulator is the hormone insulin. As your insulin levels change when you shift from the fed state to the fasted state and vice versa, your body either becomes a fat storer or a fat burner.

Now, do you see the importance of fasting and allowing your body to go into the fasted state? You may now also understand why weight-loss is one of the main benefits of intermittent fasting. Naturally, when you fast and your body burns fat, you will see those excess pounds shed effortlessly. Unlike other diets where you restrict yourself and feel bad about it, but you eat throughout the day, you might not notice yourself losing weight. Unless you give your body the chance to burn fat by "forcing" it to do so, you losing weight and maintaining a healthy weight must just be a goal, never a reality.

Of course, fat-burning and weight loss aren't the only things that occur during the fasted state. Here are other significant changes that happen in your body each time you fast:

- The levels of your growth hormones increase to promote muscle gain and fat loss.
- Your body's hormone levels adjust to accommodate the changes in body processes.
- Your metabolic rate increases, allowing you to burn more fat and calories.
- The hormone noradrenaline or norepinephrine is released. This is a fat-burning hormone.
- Your leptin levels increase. Leptin is the satiety hormone that makes you feel full.
- Your ghrelin levels decrease. Ghrelin is the hunger hormone and when you have low levels of this hormone, your appetite decreases.

The bottom line is this—your body needs the fed and fasting states to remain healthy. While we all experience these states no matter what diet we are following, intermittent fasting offers unique benefits because it lengthens the time your body remains in the fasted state. With all the good things occurring inside your body during this state, you can see why it provides so many benefits.

The Stages of Intermittent Fasting

Intermittent fasting isn't just a way to lose weight. At its best, it's a healthy lifestyle you can start following right now. Through IF, your body becomes more self-protective and efficient than it is—and all you have to do is make some modifications to your eating patterns. Just as you would advance through different stages while playing a game, IF also has different stages that you have to complete for you to move forward. As you will discover, these different stages may overlap as they don't occur at the same time or at the same rate for different people. Let's take a look at these stages:

1. **Stage 1: The Fed State (0 to 6 hours)**

   As I have mentioned, this is the stage where your insulin and blood glucose levels increase. This, in turn, stimulates the synthesis of protein so the glucose from your food goes into your cells to be utilized while any excess gets converted into glycogen and stored in the liver.

2. **Stage 2: The Fasting State (6 to 24 hours)**

When you start fasting, your insulin and blood glucose levels start to go down, and this is when your body starts burning fat for energy. When you reach 12 hours of fasting, you will be able to achieve ketosis, the process by which your body burns stored fat. Continue fasting and when you reach 18 hours, your body starts producing high levels of blood ketones. This, in turn, signals your body to increase stress-fighting pathways to improve your health. By the time you have fasted for 24 hours, a process known as autophagy occurs.

3. **Stage 3: Gluconeogenic Stage (24 to 48 hours)**

If you fast for more than 24 hours, your body would have already utilized most of your stored glycogen. This is when your body begins its transition from utilizing glucose to utilizing fat for fuel. This process may take some time and that time varies from one person to another. Ideally, while following IF, the longest time you would take to fast would be 24-hours. But let's take a look at what may happen to your body when you take things further and extend your fasting periods.

When you fast for 48 hours (2 days), your body's levels of growth hormone would go up as much as 5 times higher than when your body was in the fed state. The main reason for this elevation is that the ketones your body produces through ketosis promote the secretion of this particular hormone. The benefits of the increased growth hormone levels are a reduction of fat tissue build-up and the preservation of your lean muscle mass. It may even promote the healing of your wounds, improve your cardiovascular health, and play an important role in longevity.

Especially at the beginning, you may feel hungry during your fasting periods. But when you fast for 24 to 48 hours, expect hunger to gnaw at you more frequently and incessantly. This is a natural thing, after all, you were used to eating 3 square meals a day plus snacks. Along with these hunger pangs, you may experience a noticeable reduction in your energy levels. For some people, this also comes with irritability and a negative mood. If you plan to fast for this long, expect yourself to be more short-tempered than normal. Also, after fasting for this long, some physical changes you may experience are a lowering of your blood pressure and heart rate. While these changes might weaken your resolve to follow IF, stick with it a little longer and your body will adjust to your new eating pattern.

4. **Stage 4: Ketogenic Stage (2 to 7 days)**

After following IF for 2 to 3 days, your body enters the state of ketosis and this is when you become a fat-burning machine. Also, after 72 hours or so, your body starts breaking down aged immune cells while creating new ones to replace them. Beyond 3 days, you will start feeling a lot of changes and you will also see these changes manifest physically.

As your body remains in ketosis, you will eventually stop feeling hungry and tired. You can maintain this state by choosing the foods you eat during your feasting windows carefully. By this time, you will start losing weight mainly because your body is continuously burning your fat stores for energy. This process also has a detoxifying effect which means that your body will be cleansed of toxins. In some people, this process may have a temporary positive healing effect on their complexion.

5. **Stage 5: Mental Clarity (8 to 15 days)**

If you have finished a whole week of following your chosen IF method, congratulations! By day 8, you may start experiencing improvements in your mental clarity and mood. This is the stage that a lot of people look forward to because here, you start feeling a lot better.

Now, you may experience what some people call the "fasting high" and it typically occurs after your body has adjusted to fasting completely. Stick with it and you will notice dramatic improvements that will motivate you to keep going. These unique improvements include a restoration (or even an increase) of your energy levels, an elevation in your mood, and mental clarity.

At this stage, your body goes into a "healing mode." Your digestive system is able to take a break from the toxins and stressors it is subjected to each day. Because of this, the number of free radicals in your body goes down which, in turn, reduces your oxidative stress. While sticking with IF for this long may cause your body mild stress, this is a good thing because it makes your immune system stronger and more resilient.

6. **Stage 6: Balance and adjustment (16 days and beyond)**

By this time, you will start finding balance as your body accepts and adjusts to your new eating pattern. Your body's healing mode continues as the detoxification and healing processes continue each time you enter the fasting state. The longer your fasting states are, the more time you are providing your body with to cleanse and heal. While the beginning stages of fasting might make you feel weak and unmotivated, don't let these feelings defeat you. Just like me and all the other IF followers out there, you can push through these challenges until you can enjoy the many benefits IF has to offer.

7. **Stage 7: Refeeding (each time you break your fast)**

This is a very important stage of IF—breaking your fast—and it occurs at different times depending on the method you've chosen to follow. To help make things easier for you, it's best to break your fast with a balanced and nutrient-dense meal. This helps improve the functions of your tissues and cells further. The longer you are able to stick with your fast, the more accomplished you feel. And the more you stick with the schedule or method you have chosen, the easier your body and mind will adjust to it. At least now, you have a better idea of the different stages of IF and how you can expect to feel at each stage. You may have your own experiences at each stage but as long as you listen to your body at every turn, you may be able to reach your goals sooner than you think.

Chapter 4:

Different Types of Eating Patterns of Intermittent Fasting

Now it's time for the part that most people find interesting—learning about the different types of methods or eating patterns of IF. One great thing about IF is that it's not a strict, structured type of eating pattern where you restrict yourself too much. There are several methods you can follow and if you don't think that the one you have chosen is helping you reach your goals, change it! Naturally, those who follow a specific method will have a lot of positive things to say about that method. But if you try it and you don't think it's right for you, move on to discover the one that will benefit you the most.

Since identifying which method to use is one of the first steps on your IF journey, let me help you out with that. In this chapter, I will be sharing with you the most common methods, what they are all about, how you can start following them, and more. With this information, you will have a better idea of which methods can potentially be the next big change in your life. In other words, learning about these different methods can help you narrow down your list so you can start experimenting with them.

Flexibility is one of the greatest features of IF and you may want to take advantage of this as much as possible. By nature, intermittent fasting isn't strict so you shouldn't be too strict on yourself either. Give yourself a break and this will go a long way in maintaining your motivation until IF becomes a permanent part of your daily life.

Time-Restricted Fasting Method (16/8 or 14/10)

This type of IF method involves you selecting your own eating window each day. Ideally, you should fast between 14 to 16 hours per day to experience the benefits of IF. By the name itself, you should know that following this method means that you will restrict the time you eat so that you can stick with your fasting schedule. For this method, you can set your own fasting and feasting windows which means that you can choose a time that is most convenient for you. For instance, if you live with your family and you all have dinner at the same time, you can set your feasting window at this time. On the other hand, if you live alone, you can choose any schedule you want as long as you stick with it. Time-restricted fasting is one of the most common ways of following IF and there are a few ways to do it:

- **14:10 method**

For this method, your fasting window lasts for 14 hours while your feasting window lasts for 10 hours. For instance, you can set your eating hours between 10 in the morning and 8 in the evening each day. You can follow this schedule every day or do it a few days a week only, especially at the beginning. You also have the option to experiment with the starting time of your feasting window depending on how your daily routine goes.

- **16:8 method**

When people hear about time-restricted fasting, this is probably the method they are referring to. This is the most common IF method and it also happens to be the easiest one to follow. A lot of people also agree that this method is the most sustainable. The 16:8 method was popularized by Martin Berkhan, the fitness expert of Leangains.com, and it involves fasting for 16 hours and eating for 8 hours. Most people do this by skipping breakfast to stick with the 8-hour feasting window.

Here, you can consume around 2 to 3 meals within your fasting window. This is considered a very simple method because most people simply have an early dinner then skip breakfast the next day. This works well, especially for people who have very busy mornings. Again, you don't have to skip breakfast when following this diet. If you feel hungry in the morning or you believe that breakfast is the most important part of the day, you can start your feasting window earlier then end it earlier too as long as it only lasts for 8 hours. As with all the other methods, you can reduce your hunger by drinking a lot of water or any other type of non-caloric drinks throughout your fasting window.

- **20:4 method**

Although this is also considered a time-restricted method, it's not as common as the first two. Here, you have a longer fasting window (a whopping 20-hours) and only a 4-hour window for feasting. For most people who follow this method, they indulge themselves throughout their feasting window because they won't be able to consume excessive amounts of calories anyway. After some time, you would feel full and before you know it, your feasting window has ended.

Often, people set their feasting window in the evening, but you don't have to follow the norm. You can set it in the morning, around lunchtime or even in the afternoon. As long as you know that the time you set will allow you to eat freely and savor your meals, then that's okay. However, this method isn't ideal for beginners. You may want to start with the 14:10 or 16:8 methods first and shift to this method after your body has gotten used to the idea of fasting. As I have said, it's never a good idea to shock your body as this might be counterproductive to your health and fitness goals.

When it comes to time-restricted fasting, your start time doesn't really matter. But it's recommended to have the same start time each day as this will help you build a routine for your body to adjust easily. Interestingly, I have also read a lot of sources that recommend women only fast for 14 to 15 hours to stay healthy. That's definitely something to think about when choosing which method to follow.

24-Hour Fasting Method

This IF method is also known as the "eat-stop-eat" method and it was made popular by Brad Pilon, another fitness expert. For this method, you would fast for a whole day—or 24 hours—either 1 or 2 times each week. This method of fasting isn't for the faint of heart, as 24 hours is quite a long time. If it's your first time fasting, you may want to try the other methods first before you switch to this one. The 24-hour fasting method isn't the best place to start as longer fasts can be more challenging.

Among all the different fasting methods, this one is fairly simple. For instance, at the start of the week (Monday), you finish your dinner at 8:00 in the evening. Then you wouldn't eat anything until 8:00 in the evening the next day (Tuesday). Basically, you would break your fast at the same time you started fasting the day before. You can do this at any time of the day. Like all other fasting windows, you can consume non-caloric beverages to ease your hunger, but you shouldn't eat any solids.

It's important to note that this method involves a 24-hour fast only. This means that you should eat the day before and the day after your fasting day. Extending your fast isn't recommended, especially if you're a beginner. That's why this method only involves fasting for 1 to 2 times a week. Some health experts say that this is a very effective method of losing weight because fat-burning is at its peak somewhere between the 16th and 24th fasting hours. This means that if you follow this method, there is a very high likelihood that you would experience this benefit. But if you want to follow the 24-hour fasting method to shed excess pounds, make sure that you eat normally on days when you aren't fasting. By this, I mean that you would eat the same way as you would if you weren't fasting. Don't try to compensate for the food you didn't eat for 24 hours or you might end up seeing the opposite results.

If you try this method and you feel that it works well for you, then you may extend your fast to 36 hours (1 1/2 days). For most people who do this, their purpose is to either force their body into ketosis or to reach a deeper state of ketosis. However, it isn't recommended to do this frequently. If you would like to push yourself, you may do this once a week or once a month just to enhance the benefits.

Somewhat related to this method is another IF method known as One Meal A Day or OMAD. This is one of the more extreme IF methods that I wouldn't recommend for beginners either. Here, you would only have one meal each day, every day. I say that it's related to the 24-hour fasting method because you would eat one meal then wait 24 hours before eating your next meal. However, for this method, you would be doing this daily. If you plan to follow this method, prepare yourself as it will test your spirit and your mind. Also, if you want to follow OMAD (after you have tried the casier methods first), make sure to plan your meal well as this is where you will be getting all of your nutrients. Make sure that you eat a balanced and healthy meal each day so that you don't end up developing deficiencies. Furthermore, make sure that you don't overeat as this is not a healthy habit you should develop as part of your intermittent fasting lifestyle.

5:2 Fasting Method

For this IF method, the numbers don't refer to the hours of your feasting and fasting. Instead, they refer to the number of days. The 5:2 fasting method was developed by Dr. Michael Mosley who is also a British journalist. Here, you would only consume 500 to 600 calories for 2 days (non-consecutive) and eat normally on the other 5 days. This is a unique method as you won't fast completely, you would only reduce your caloric intake drastically on the 2 days.

While this method can help you lose weight too, the benefits aren't as pronounced as the other methods. If you're on the fence about IF or you feel overwhelmed with the concept of fasting, you may start with this method. It's easier to follow and it allows you to ease into intermittent fasting to give your body time to get used to not eating as much or as frequently as you are now.

If you plan to follow this diet, choose two non-consecutive days each week where you will restrict your caloric intake. While you don't have to set a fasting window during these days, you can either spread out the 500 to 600 calories by eating small meals throughout the day or you can also consume one big meal amounting to the same amount of calories. For the rest of the 5 days, you can eat normally. Again, don't overeat and don't try to compensate. Just eat as you normally would, to make it easier for you to adjust.

Warrior Fasting Method

Another fitness expert, this time by the name of Ori Hofmekler, developed and popularized this diet. Simply put, it involves fasting throughout the day and eating one huge meal at night. While it may seem a lot like the OMAD method, there are some differences. For one, you are allowed to consume minimal amounts of raw vegetables and fruits throughout the day instead of sticking with non-caloric beverages only.

Following this method is another way for you to enjoy the benefits of IF. Unlike the other methods, this one has a relatively interesting origin. Hormelker used to be a member of the Israeli Special Force and he developed the diet to mimic the diet of warriors during ancient times. Apparently, the warriors during those times were able to maintain slim waistlines and sharp minds by eating minimal amounts throughout the day and consuming a huge meal come night time. In other words, your fasting window would be the whole day plus the time you sleep at night while your feasting window would be set at night and you give yourself a maximum of 4 hours to eat all you need. This method was one of the first methods that became popular among all the other IF methods.

Are you familiar with the paleo diet? If not, you may want to read about it if you plan to follow this method. I mention this diet because the Warrior fasting method highlights food options that are similar to the ones emphasized on the paleo diet. This means that you should opt for whole and unprocessed foods when preparing your meals. If you're already on paleo, then combining it with this IF method will do wonders for your health.

Also, if you plan to follow this method, you have the option to fast for the whole day (meaning, you won't eat anything, not even raw veggies and fruits) and have your large, nutrient-dense meal at night. But when you're starting out, you may want to indulge in the snacks that you are "allowed" to eat at night. Again, this will make it easier to adjust compared to foregoing solid food altogether. Also, enjoying small, healthy snacks throughout the day can prevent you from overeating at night as well as prevent indigestion and other stomach issues.

Alternate-Day Fasting Method

Here's another simple method of IF for you to follow and it's similar to the 5:2 method. The name itself suggests that alternate-day fasting involves fasting every other day. Unlike other methods, this one comes with a number of versions. If this is your first time fasting, try not to fast completely every other day. If you do, you will end up feeling very hungry at least 3 times a week. As I have experienced, this isn't a pleasant feeling and it made me stop after just 2 weeks.

A nutrition professor named Krista Varady, Ph.D. from the University of Illinois popularized this method. While this is one of the more popular IF methods out there, you may want to ease into it before going all out. This means that you eat normally on alternate days while reducing your caloric intake on the other days. For instance, you can eat normally for 4 days (Monday, Wednesday, Friday, and Sunday) while reducing your daily caloric intake to 20% on alternate days (Tuesday, Thursday, and Saturday). Either way, this method makes it easier for you because you are able to eat normally for a number of days before reducing your caloric intake. This intermittent method will kick start your metabolism to improve its functions.

Starting the alternate-day fasting method this way makes it less challenging. By the second week, you may notice that you don't feel as hungry as when you first started. By the fourth week, you may feel more satisfied with this method of eating. While this method isn't for me, it might be the one you feel most comfortable with. As I said, it's all about trying the different methods to see which one works for your own lifestyle. One thing you should know about this method is that since it's quite intense, a lot of people don't think that it is sustainable in the long-term.

Short-Term vs. Long-Term Fasting Periods

Now that you know more about the most common IF methods, you may already start thinking about which one(s) to try out. The important thing is to ease into IF instead of trying to do too much, too fast. Remember, your aim is to make IF part of your life. You shouldn't push yourself into fasting just because you want to experience all the benefits right away. Besides, most of the benefits only come after your body has adjusted to this new eating pattern and you are following the method you have chosen consistently. The fact is, there is a difference between short-term and long-term fasting. For instance, while short-term fasting is easier, long-term fasting may come with more benefits. Let's dive into the definitions and benefits of these fasts to help clear some important things up.

Long-term fasting

Long-term fasts come in different forms, some of which can be quite dangerous. For instance, there is a method known as a "dry fast" that doesn't permit you to eat anything, not even water. This can cause harm to you as it's not recommended to go for more than 24 hours without drinking anything. Then there is water fasting where you only drink water and nothing else. Juice fasting, on the other hand, is where you would only consume fresh vegetable and fruit juices. Some even fast by only consuming low-calorie protein mixes or broths. Here are some benefits long-term fasts like these have to offer.

1. **Weight loss**

Naturally, when you don't consume food for long periods of time or you restrict yourself severely, you will lose a lot of weight. In fact, the longer you stick with these fasts, the faster you will be able to shed your excess weight. For the more extreme types of fasts (like water fasts or dry fasts), you may lose 1 to 2 pounds a day. However, doing this for a long time might end up making you sick. Also, as soon as you stop fasting and you go back to your old diet, there is a high possibility of gaining back all the weight you had lost.

2. Autophagy

I have already explained what autophagy is, right? If you recall, this is a cleansing process for your cells. This is one of the best benefits of fasting no matter what method you use. Apart from helping you reach a healthy weight, autophagy also has powerful muscle-building and anti-aging benefits.

3. Helps you break bad eating habits

Another benefit you may enjoy from long-term fasting is that it can help you get rid of your bad eating habits such as emotional eating, overeating, binge eating, and more. As long as you have done research about the fasting method you choose (unless it's intermittent fasting), you can improve your life by learning some new, healthier eating habits. However, if you allow yourself to make up for everything or compensate for all the time you fasted each time you eat, then you won't be able to break these habits. If you plan to make fasting part of your life, you must make a conscious effort to change and break these habits.

As with any other diet or eating plan, there are some precautions you need to take for long-term fasting. First of all, make sure that you are healthy enough to embark on such a change. You can do this by going to your doctor and talking to them about your plans. If you suffer from any kind of medical condition, think twice about long-term fasting. You don't want to risk worsening your condition just so you can enjoy the potential benefits fasting has to offer. Do research, make a realistic plan, and always put your own health and safety first.

Short-term fasting

This type of fasting is where IF falls into. IF is classified as a short-term fasting method because the different methods only recommend that you fast for a specific amount of time and only as much as 24-hours. Despite this, a lot of people may find it a challenge to restrict their daily food intake consistently. Yes, it's challenging. But as I and many others have proved, it's not impossible. And the great thing about short-term fasting is that it may provide a lot of the same benefits without having to go extreme or restricting yourself to the point that you end up feeling miserable.

In Chapter 2, we had already discussed the different benefits of IF and most of these apply to other short-term fasting methods, too. To help you remember, here are some of the best benefits this type of fasting has to offer:

- It promotes autophagy, the process that cleanses the body of defective and damaged parts of your cells.
- It may help prevent or reduce the risk of developing cancer.
- It promotes the health of the brain along with the functions and structure.
- It may help reduce the risk of heart disease by reducing the risk factors.
- It may improve longevity because of all the other health.

Do you remember all of these and more? You may go back to the second chapter to recall all of these benefits and remember how they affect your body. While IF isn't perfect, it does seem like the better option. It can provide you with a number of restorative and preventive functions that contribute to your overall health. Therefore, if you're at the peak of your health and you want to improve your life even further, this is another reason for you to try IF.

No matter what type of fasting you plan to try, you must learn how to listen to your body. Since you will be making a significant change in your eating habits, you will definitely start experiencing some changes. If these changes are good, keep going. But if something doesn't feel right, you fall ill or you feel like your existing condition is getting worse, stop. Never force yourself to follow IF or any other kind of diet. Don't worry, I will explain to you the potential risks of IF along with the precautions to take before ending this book. That way, you get a complete picture of what IF really is and how you can start following it in the safest possible way.

Chapter 5

Making Intermittent Fasting Part of Your Lifestyle

Now that all the basic and technical information is out of the way, I hope you gained a more profound understanding of what intermittent fasting is. We have already gone through the definition, benefits, and even the different methods of IF. With everything you have learned so far, you should already have a stronger urge to start following this unique but beneficial eating pattern.

When it comes to making IF part of your life, you must first create your own routine to make the diet more manageable. This, in turn, increases the likelihood that you will stick with IF for the foreseeable future. Sticking with this eating pattern will ensure that you will experience long-term health benefits. And the longer your body adjusts to IF, the more confidently you can "level-up" by easing yourself into the more complex or challenging methods. Intimidating as IF may seem, it's actually quite easy.

One of the best things that I love about IF is the fact that I don't have to focus too much on what I eat. Personally, I have found that changing my eating schedule or eating habits is a lot easier than trying to restrict myself from eating certain types of foods or food groups. As I have already started my own IF journey and I've been on it for some time now, I have a lot of things to share with you. Here, I will share with you some tips, pointers, and strategies that have worked wonders for me and for other IF enthusiasts I know. As you go through these pointers, you can do your own experimentation to see which ones work for you so you can come up with your own plan of action.

The Simplicity of IF

Apart from all the health benefits intermittent fasting has to offer, another key benefit of IF is that it simplifies your life. Once you establish your routine, you will discover that IF is easy to maintain as it takes away a lot of the demands in terms of your eating habits. You don't have to count calories, prepare 3 meals a day plus snacks, think about what to eat for all of these meals, and more.

The simplicity of IF is one of the reasons why it's becoming more popular with people all over the world. Fasting has been an existing concept since the beginning and now, health and fitness experts have refined the practice to make it more accessible and easier for us to follow. The fact that IF has different variations makes it even more appealing because you don't have to stick with a single standard diet that comes with strict rules and guidelines.

Simple as IF is, it's a flexible eating plan that is incredibly effective at helping people lose weight. As with most IF enthusiasts, this was one of the reasons why I became interested in following this trendy eating pattern. And after trying different diets without seeing myself progress toward my health and fitness goals, I am glad that this one caught my interest. Now, here I am sharing everything I had learned to help you and countless others make the choice to follow IF in the long-term. As long as you follow the method you have chosen properly, IF can be a powerful tool for you to become healthier and happier overall. With that being said, let's move on to how you can follow IF correctly.

Establishing IF as Part of Your Lifestyle

I wrote this book to help people like you make IF part of your lifestyle. The easiest way to do this is by making it more manageable. That way, you can start forming long-term, healthy habits to enjoy ongoing benefits. While all of the pointers that I will share with you can help you out, you should also come up with your own personal approach. Ease into the diet and take an incremental approach rather than pushing yourself too hard.

First of all, you must manage your expectations. While IF can be very effective and beneficial to your health, you shouldn't focus on all this right away. Otherwise, you might get disappointed because you don't see immediate results. Because of this, you might lose your motivation then give up before you can see any good changes. Once you have made the choice to follow IF, your first goal should be to get yourself (and your body) used to the new changes. Find the best method that will make you feel good about following IF instead of trying to see the results right away.

This is why I jumped from one method to another. While I went into this journey feeling positive and motivated, the first method I picked didn't really make me feel that great. So I kept trying until I discovered the method that worked best for me. I focused on myself and listened to what my body was telling me. Then I worked on making the schedule part of my routine and refining my diet to bring balance to my life. Here are some practical tips and strategies to help you establish IF in your own life:

1. **As much as possible, strive for a clean diet**

While IF doesn't come with guidelines about what foods to eat and what foods to avoid, this doesn't mean that you should only eat processed, junk, or packaged foods during your feasting window. If you really want to improve your health and enjoy all the benefits of IF, try to strive for a cleaner diet. If you are used to those "unhealthy" options, try reducing your intake gradually. You don't have to eliminate them altogether, just opt for healthier choices whenever possible.

In the past, you may have gotten used to eating junk food for your snack while enjoying healthy, balanced meals for breakfast, lunch, and dinner. But once you start IF, you won't be eating as frequently as before. If you get rid of your healthy, balanced meals and keep the unhealthy snacks, this will result in poor health. Over time, you might even develop deficiencies. I'm not saying that you should rid yourself of these tasty but unhealthy treats. Just try to focus more on giving your body all the nutrients it requires to remain healthy and function well. While following IF, the cleaner your diet is, the faster your body will adjust.

2. Don't let hunger bring you down

No matter what IF method you choose, expect to feel hungry at some point. This is especially true if you have never tried fasting in the past. In fact, in the beginning, you may feel like you are always hungry. Instead of allowing this to bring you down, try to anticipate this feeling and embrace it when it comes. Accept the fact that this is one of the toughest parts of IF, but know that you will get through it.

Difficult as this may be, it will take a lot of willpower and mental strength to get through the first few days or weeks of intermittent fasting. To stick with it and motivate yourself, try to remember your reasons for following IF along with the health and fitness goals you want to achieve. If you need to, distract yourself from the hunger you feel instead of giving in to it. Don't worry too much. As time goes by, you will get used to skipping meals and surviving without eating for hours at a time.

3. **Don't go overboard when your feasting window comes**

As your fasting window comes to an end, you will feel excited at the thought of eating and satisfying your hunger. This is understandable, I've been there too. However, one of the easiest mistakes you can make is thinking that you can eat as much as you want and whatever you want during your feasting window. But it's not like that.

When your feasting window comes, try to restrain yourself and stick with a reasonable amount of food. Whether you plan to eat one big meal or a few small meals throughout your fasting window, try not to go overboard. Ideally, you should be at a caloric deficit, especially if you want to lose weight. Overeating is easy, but it's not right. Use your willpower to restrain yourself until you notice that you are getting used to your new eating pattern.

4. Consider working out while fasting

For this tip, you can take it as a friendly suggestion. In the long run, it will help you focus on other things instead of your hungry feelings. If you already have a workout routine, the best time to do it is during your fasting window. Otherwise, you would be taking precious time away from your feasting window. Also, it's never a good idea to work out right after eating meals.

You may be wondering how you can possibly workout when you don't have food in your tummy. Don't worry about this, because our bodies are genetically wired to provide you with energy even while you're in a fasted state. As a matter of fact, when you work out while fasting, this helps give your energy levels a boost. Not only that, you can enjoy a sharper and clearer mind too when you exercise during your fasting window. Just don't overdo it, especially at the beginning.

If working out isn't a part of your daily routine, you may want to consider it. After all, regular exercise offers a lot of benefits. Combine this with your healthy new eating pattern and you're sure to start seeing all the good benefits in no time!

Where to Start

After reading about the different IF methods, have you decided which one to start with? A lot of people start with time-restricted methods like 16:8 or 14:10 as these are quite easy to get used to. Whether you plan to start with this method or any of the other ones, start off slowly and build-up incrementally over time. For instance, if you plan to follow the 16:8 method, you can start off with short fasting windows. As your body adjusts, you can lengthen your fasting time until you are able to reach 16 hours. Keep increasing the time you fast as comfort allows. Here are a few more pointers for you to help you start following IF:

- **Speak with your doctor**

Whether you're at the peak of your health or you are suffering from any kind of medical condition, getting the green light from your doctor is very important. Intermittent fasting is a big change, especially if you have no experience of fasting in the past. Since IF is trending right now, there is a high likelihood that your doctor already knows about it and they may even have valuable advice for you to help you follow it. This is one thing I had done before following IF and my doctor was all for it. Getting your doctor's approval is one of the safest ways for you to start on IF.

- **Establish your health goals**

Most people who choose to follow IF do so because they want to reach certain goals. Weight loss is one of the most common goals, but you may have your own health goals in mind. After going through the benefits of IF, you can see whether or not this eating pattern will help you reach your goals. But since you're already in this part of the book, that means that your mind is already set on IF.

This tip is very important since it will help you customize your own IF plan. For instance, if your main goal is to lose weight, choose an IF method that will help you achieve this. Even if you have to work your way through different methods, as long as you have your goal(s) in mind, this gives your efforts a purpose. Besides, goals can be very powerful motivators.

- **Choose your IF method**

Next up, choose the IF method to follow. As I have mentioned earlier and as per experience, you can choose a few options and try them out first to see if they work for you. The great thing about IF is that it offers flexibility. When you're starting out, you don't have to follow all the rules of the methods right away. Also, you can focus on learning how to fast and helping your body adjust to this practice first before you start cleaning up your diet.

The tip I shared in the last section about choosing healthy options makes IF more sustainable, but you don't have to start it right away (unless you want to). After you have chosen your IF method, plan your schedule and try to stick with it as much as possible. Then when it's time for you to eat, you can eat the foods that will make you feel happy and satisfied. When you feel like your body has already gotten used to fasting and you want to level-up, then you can start making adjustments to your diet to make it cleaner, healthier, and more balanced.

- **Observe your body for any changes and learn how to listen**

Even if you're a spontaneous kind of person, when it comes to making changes to your diet, this is one time when you may want to slow down a bit. Take things one step at a time to ensure better results. Think about it—what will happen to your body if you suddenly fast for 24 hours without preparing for it? Chances are, you will experience weakening, extreme hunger, and other adverse side effects.

After choosing your IF method, learn everything you can about it. Then make a plan for how you will follow it for the next few days, weeks, or months. One thing I have learned is that when you start with smaller fasting windows, this helps you stick with your eating schedule more. For instance, if you decide to start by fasting for 10 hours including your sleeping time, this means that you would only have to fast for about 2 to 4 hours a day depending on how many hours you sleep each night.

On the other hand, if you immediately fast for 16 hours, this means that you would have to fast between 8 to 10 hours a day. If you're not used to fasting, there is a very high likelihood that you would end up breaking your fast. I'm not saying this is a bad thing, especially in the beginning. Listening to your body means that when you're hungry and you can't take it anymore, eat something. Don't allow yourself to suffer as this will de-motivate you. When you listen to your body and observe the changes happening, this makes your experience a more positive one. This, in turn, inspires you to keep going until you reach your goals.

- **Keep track of your progress**

There are many ways for you to monitor your progress while following IF and it's best to do this from the very beginning. Personally, I kept a journal where I wrote down all of the emotional and physical observations I had. In the same journal, I also kept track of my weight (since weight loss was one of my goals). If you're not a fan of keeping a journal, you can come up with your own method for monitoring your progress. The important thing here is that you keep track of everything as this will make you feel more motivated and accountable.

While keeping track of your progress, you will also be able to determine whether the method you have chosen is working for you or not. Through the data you gather about yourself, you can make adjustments to your plans as needed. Give yourself enough time to adjust and when you feel like you need to skip one or two fasting sessions, don't stress over it. Adhering rigidly to the schedule you have chosen will decrease the sustainability of your new eating pattern. But by not pushing yourself too hard, you will be able to establish healthier habits that will last for a long time.

Implementing a Program

Part of planning your IF journey is coming up with a program or schedule. This serves as a guide for you. Coming up with a schedule allows you to incorporate your new eating pattern into your life. This makes it more conducive for you to start learning new, healthier habits. Following a schedule enables you to practice consistency which, in turn, makes it easier for you to form a regular routine.

Some methods of intermittent fasting allow you to consume healthy foods during your fasting windows. However, most of them recommend that you fast completely from solid foods and liquids that contain calories. These are little things you must remember depending on the method you have chosen to follow. Now, let's go through some helpful guidelines for you as you create a plan to implement for your intermittent fasting journey:

- **Take IF on as a new habit instead of a temporary fix**

  If you haven't been following any kind of diet, then you're probably used to eating 3 square meals a day with a few snacks in between. Because of this, prepare yourself to feel uneasy as you try fasting for the first time. For instance, if you set the start of your fasting window before dinner all the way to breakfast, you will have the urge to eat come dinner time. This is one of the most challenging parts of intermittent fasting. But when you think about it, breaking any habit and creating a new one always comes with a challenge, right?

As you start on IF, think of it as learning a new habit. Give your body and mind time to get accustomed to the new eating pattern and the schedule you set for yourself. Prepare yourself mentally for this change and this will increase your chances of success. Stay firm, remain flexible, and have fun with it.

- **In the beginning, keep your fasting periods short**

In the beginning, one of your main goals should be to get yourself used to fasting. With short fasting windows, you won't feel as overwhelmed or as hungry as you would if you start off with longer fasting windows. Take it easy on yourself and as you fast, try to observe how you are feeling. This allows you to better determine whether you can already lengthen your fasting hours or not.

When you immediately fast for a long time, you may experience a number of side effects like inability to focus, dehydration (especially if you don't drink enough calorie-free liquids), irritability, other changes in your mood, low levels of energy, and more. As soon as you are feeling severe symptoms, it's recommended to stop. If you do, don't beat yourself up over it. We've all been there, we've all experienced giving it to our hunger because it was accompanied by worrying symptoms. Learn from all of your experiences and this will help you become wiser and more effective in terms of fasting.

- **Drink to ease your hunger**

Intermittent fasting isn't like dry fasting where you shouldn't consume anything. During your fasting windows, you can ease your hunger by drinking water, coffee, tea, and other beverages without calories. These will keep you hydrated and will give you some sense of fullness to distract you from the hunger you're feeling. Remember, hunger is natural so don't surrender to it right away.

- **Try different things**

Intermittent fasting comes with recommended rules for you to follow. These rules and guidelines will help you follow the method you have chosen correctly which, in turn, allows you to enjoy the benefits of IF after following it for some time. But what sets IF apart from other diets (aside from the fact that IF isn't really a type of diet) is that you don't have to follow strict rules.

For instance, the method I am following now works well for me and for other people, but it might not be right for you. Or some of the strategies I have shared here may have done wonders for my IF journey, but you might not be too keen on following them. You can think of IF as a customizable eating pattern and you can find what works best for you by trying different things.

- **Know what you're allowed to consume**

One of the most dangerous misconceptions about IF is that you can eat absolutely anything during your feasting window. After all, it's called a "feasting window" for a reason, right?

Wrong.

I have already emphasized the importance of not overeating during your feasting window. Apart from this, it's also recommended to avoid highly processed food along with foods that are either too sugary or salty, junk food, and other types of unhealthy food items. You don't have to eliminate these from your diet right away, but don't binge on these types of food either. Instead, focus on healthier options that are tasty, too. That way, you can enjoy your eating time while still ensuring your health.

Beverages are easier during your feasting window because you can drink practically anything. Just try not to overindulge on beverages that contain high amounts of sugar so you don't mess up your insulin levels too much. During your fasting window, the reason why you should only drink non-caloric beverages is because these don't trigger the release of insulin in your body. Therefore, drinking these beverages doesn't interfere with autophagy or ketosis.

- **Find ways to keep yourself motivated**

As you come up with a plan for your intermittent fasting journey, try to think of ways to keep yourself motivated throughout. For instance, I set weekly mini-goals for myself. I made sure that these goals were easy, realistic, but also provided enough of a challenge. Each time I was able to reach these goals, I felt motivated to keep going. Since you know yourself well, you can come up with these motivational methods and include them in your plans. While not directly related to IF, this is a very important tip for you.

- **Learn how to strategize**

By now, I have already shared with you a lot of strategies, tips, and pointers to help you succeed. Some of these may work well for you while others won't. Therefore, you should also try to come up with your own strategies to deal with the challenges of IF and strengthen your willpower.

For instance, although there isn't any requirement for the time to start fasting or feasting, it's interesting to note that nighttime eating is commonly associated with the risk of diabetes and obesity. If you want to lose weight or you have a history of diabetes, then you may want to set your feasting window sometime during the day.

You can also ask your doctor about taking vitamins or supplements while on IF to make sure that you don't end up deficient in any nutrient. You also have the option to count your calories (this isn't one of the rules, but it can be very helpful), especially if weight loss is one of your goals. Now, try to think of other strategies you can use to improve your chances of success. Along the way, you can come up with these strategies as you encounter challenges and other interesting experiences while you follow the IF method you've chosen.

Addressing the Urge to Eat

The first time you try fasting, you will feel things that you have never experienced in the past. The first time you feel hungry while fasting, ask yourself if you're really hungry or if it's just an impulse because you normally eat at this time. As you follow IF, you should be able to distinguish between physical hunger, cravings, contextual prompts, and learned routines. As you feel "hunger," try pushing your boundaries a bit further without being too rigid or being too hard on yourself. Then try to observe how you feel after this gentle push.

Going to bed hungry is never a good feeling. Trying to accomplish your tasks while feeling hungry isn't fun either. And for some people, it may take up to a week or more to adjust to their new pattern of eating. Hunger is an inevitable part of intermittent fasting, but it doesn't have to be the thing that defeats you. While anticipating hunger is helpful, dreading it isn't something you should be doing. After all, hunger is a transient feeling and it only lasts for about 20 minutes or so. Surprising, isn't it? A lot of people don't know this because they tend to satisfy their hunger as soon as they can.

When it comes to hunger, the best advice I can give you is to understand that feeling hungry is okay. Uncomfortable as hunger is, it's just a temporary thing and nothing bad will happen to you because of it. To help you address your hunger and the urge to eat that comes with it, here are some things to try:

- **Learn how to manage your stress and always try to get enough sleep each night**

  High levels of stress and poor sleeping habits have a powerful effect on your appetite. This is mainly because they disrupt your blood sugar and hormone levels. To avoid hunger pangs caused by these imbalances, learn how to manage your stress more effectively. There are plenty of stress reduction techniques you can try to help avoid stress eating.

Getting enough sleep each night will also help curb your stress, as well as your hunger. To improve the quality of your sleep, make sure that your bedroom is well-ventilated and cool enough for you to sleep comfortably. Try to sleep and wake up at roughly the same time each night and every morning. Come up with your own bedtime routine to make it easier for you to fall asleep and stay asleep throughout the night.

- **Opt for high-fat, low-carb food options**

After adjusting to your new eating pattern, it's time to make a few changes in your diet. While these changes aren't required, choosing high-fat, low-carb options allow you to get the most out of your feasting window. These types of foods promote satiety, stabilize your blood sugar levels, and make fasting easier.

- **Learn how to differentiate physical hunger**

and psychological hunger

According to researchers, there are certain cells in our stomach responsible for regulating the release of ghrelin, the hormone associated with hunger and appetite. The cells responsible for producing this hormone have their own circadian rhythms that synchronize our anticipation of food with our body's metabolic cycles. This means that eating 3 meals a day (breakfast, lunch, and dinner) is actually a learned or trained behavior. Often, when you feel "hungry" in the morning, it's because you know that it's time for you to eat. But this hunger you feel might not be physical hunger. Instead, it's all in your mind. Once you are able to understand and accept this, dealing with your hunger becomes easier.

- **Make sure that you are well-hydrated during your fasting window**

Often, when you feel thirsty, you confuse this with hunger. So if you make sure that you're always well-hydrated, you won't have to deal with this confusing feeling. In the morning, try to drink 1 to 2 glasses of water as soon as you wake up. Throughout the day, try to drink at least 2 liters of water. Just don't go overboard as drinking too much will flush out your electrolytes.

Apart from keeping you healthy, drinking a lot of water will help you feel full so you don't experience a lot of hunger pangs. Of course, water isn't the only option you have while fasting. You can also drink other liquids as long as they don't contain any calories. These will also give you a feeling of fullness along with the satisfaction of consuming something to quell your hunger.

One beverage you should try to limit or avoid is alcohol. This is especially important right before you fast. Drinking alcohol can mess up your blood sugar and hormone levels. This makes it more difficult to fast. If you still want to have a drink before fasting, stick to low-carb alcoholic drinks and don't drink excessive amounts.

- **Increase your salt intake and replace your electrolytes**

One common side effect of intermittent fasting is the loss of electrolytes. When this happens, you may feel thirsty more frequently and you might even develop dry mouth. Aside from being uncomfortable, these symptoms will make you feel hungry too. You can overcome this issue by adding more salt to your meals and drinking bone broth during your feasting windows. You may also consider taking potassium and magnesium supplements as these can help replenish your electrolytes as well.

- **Distract yourself from your hunger**

If you start feeling hungry and you just sit there wallowing in your hunger, you'll end up feeling miserable. As you are training yourself to eat at different times of the day, distract yourself from your hunger. For instance, if lunchtime is approaching and you are still fasting, find something to do. Take a walk outside, read a book, go for a jog, and more. Try to find activities that are enjoyable for you so you don't end up thinking about food while doing them. Don't allow yourself to be idle or bored so you don't focus on your hunger too much.

All of these tips and the ones you come up with on your own will help you cast your hunger aside and get used to fasting for hours at a time. Let me remind you once again, just don't be too strict or too hard on yourself. If you think that you really can't take it anymore and your hunger is starting to take a toll on your body, eat something healthy. But if you feel like you can push through your hunger, go for it!

The Importance of Self-Compassion on IF

Have you ever tried starting a diet before?

Personally, I have tried following different kinds of diets in the past, but to no avail. One of the biggest mistakes I've made in the past is being too harsh on myself. When I tried following restrictive diets, I frequently ended up eating the foods I should have been avoiding...then I felt guilty after. This is one of the reasons why I never really found success in such diets. Back then, I never practiced self-compassion. Maybe if I did, I would have been able to stick with dieting.

Practicing self-compassion helps increase your resilience which, in turn, increases the likelihood that you will stick with intermittent fasting. Being more compassionate with yourself improves the sustainability of IF instead of being too rigid or too harsh on yourself when you make a mistake. After all, if you miss a day or two, that won't really undo all the efforts you have already put into the diet. Neither will this halt all the potential benefits of IF. You can think of self-compassion as your secret weapon in getting rid of your negative attitude towards dieting to improve your chances of success.

Basically, self-compassion means that you treat yourself with the same compassion as you would toward other people. Self-compassion has 3 important elements that you should understand:

1. **Common humanity**

Most people have a "dieting mindset" where they believe that when they fail, they're the only ones. Does this sound familiar to you? I had this mindset in the past and it was very self-defeating. When you think this way, you end up believing that you don't have enough willpower and you're getting everything wrong as you try to start a diet or eating plan. While you may think that you're the only one who feels this way, you're not. Almost all people have the same mindset.

When you make a mistake, try not to think that you failed. You are not the only one who has experienced challenges while starting IF (or any other type of diet for that matter). Be more compassionate with yourself by connecting with others who share the same struggles as you. If needed, join IF groups or communities and connect with others who are on the same journey. Apart from everything you learn from this book, you may also learn a lot from them while learning how to be more compassionate with yourself, too.

2. Mindfulness

When you have negative thoughts or feelings about your new eating pattern, don't let these define you. You don't have to repress or deny these negativities. Instead, accept them, try to learn from them, and know that these will all pass. By practicing mindfulness, you will be able to change your relationship with food and transform it into a more positive one. You will also be able to handle your emotions more effectively which, in turn, can help you stick with intermittent fasting easily, too.

3. Self-kindness

Throughout your journey, there will be a lot of times when you would talk to yourself. To keep yourself motivated by practicing self-compassion, make sure that whenever you do self-talk, you are always kind. Self-kindness is very important as this will make the whole experience more positive. Keep convincing yourself that you are strong enough and that you can handle all the challenges that come with IF. One day you'll come to realize that you don't just believe what you are saying, but you have already achieved what you are trying to convince yourself of.

Practicing self-compassion makes you less judgmental towards yourself. This is essential if you want to make IF a permanent part of your lifestyle. Aside from this, the practice also offers a number of benefits including:

- It improves your emotional and mental health which, in turn, helps strengthen your resolve.
- It makes you more accepting of yourself so you can deal with challenges and difficulties more effectively.
- It promotes a healthier relationship with food. This is especially important if you have a lot of issues when it comes to dieting and you want to overcome them once and for all.

Just like any other practice, using self-compassion frequently will make it stronger. This isn't something that comes naturally, you have to consciously work on it. The more you do, the more it can become a powerful tool for your IF success. It helps you move forward no matter what comes your way by empowering you and increasing your belief in your own capabilities.

Chapter 6

The Risks, Side Effects, and Precautions of Intermittent Fasting

Throughout this book, I have explained to you how great intermittent fasting is and how much it has changed my life for the better. Of course, as someone who has experienced the benefits of this unique eating pattern firsthand, I have a lot of good things to say about it. But this doesn't mean that I think it's the perfect diet for anyone. I've also shared how I struggled with IF, especially at the beginning. I wasn't one of those people who was able to pick a method and realize that it was the perfect one for me.

Apart from that, I had also experienced the difficulties of adjusting to the new eating pattern I subjected myself to, especially at the beginning. The point that I am trying to share here is that intermittent fasting isn't perfect. Yes, it's doable. Yes, it's legit. But it also comes with its own risks and precautions.

If you've ever tried doing a search for intermittent fasting online, you will come across hundreds of thousands of resources on it. Unfortunately, not everything you will find online is accurate. There is a lot of misinformation surrounding this trendy new eating pattern and this adds to the confusion people feel about it. By now, you already know the good things about IF. I've even shared with you several practical tips and strategies that you can use to help you and guide you as you start your IF journey. But before you make the final choice to follow IF and before you start making your plans, let me show you the other side of the coin.

While intermittent fasting doesn't have a "dark side" or something equally sinister, it does come with its own risks. Knowing these risks will allow you to make a more solid decision on whether IF is right for you or not. In this chapter, that is exactly what you are going to learn about. By the end of this chapter, you will have a clearer and more complete picture of IF. Only then can you make your final choice.

Precautions: What You Need to Know Before Starting IF

Before reading this book, you may have thought that IF was a technical or complicated thing. But now that you understand it more, you know that it's as simple as cycling between periods of eating and periods of not eating (fasting). Aside from the fact that fasting as a practice has been around since ancient times, it isn't something new to any of us either. Think about it—you don't really eat at every moment throughout the day, right? After having breakfast, you go about your day until it's time to have lunch. The time you spend without eating between your first meal of the day and your second meal of the day is already time spent fasting. Throughout the day, you already have short fasts wherein you do other things aside from eating.

It's that simple.

This means that when you decide to follow an intermittent fasting method, you would just lengthen your fasting periods. Despite all the benefits of IF and the popular belief these days, intermittent fasting isn't suitable for everyone. Even though there are different methods to choose from, IF isn't a "one-size-fits-all" diet or eating plan. That's why I recommended that you speak with your doctor first before trying it out.

Remember that although there have been a lot of animal studies done on IF and its benefits, further research is needed to prove that all of these benefits also apply to humans. Right now, we mostly rely on anecdotal reports and our own experiences after following IF for some time. Apart from studying the benefits, researchers should also conduct more studies about the potential risks or side effects of this eating plan. Having concrete evidence about the benefits and risks of IF makes it a lot easier to decide whether you should follow it or not.

When you are healthy and you are looking for a new way to improve your health further, IF could be an excellent choice. However, health practitioners and experts claim that certain people shouldn't consider IF or any other form of fasting. If you fall into any of these groups of people, you shouldn't continue with IF, or you should consult with your doctor first and get the green light before you start:

- **If you're pregnant, breastfeeding, or trying to conceive**

  If you're trying to conceive, it's not a good idea to start a new diet. To increase your chances of getting pregnant, you should be at the peak of your health. You should also follow a healthy, balanced diet to make it easier.

Once you get pregnant, fasting isn't a good idea either because you have extra energy needs. You will be growing a person inside you and that person needs to be nourished, not deprived of food. Remember, when you fast, so will the fetus growing inside you. Even after giving birth, if you plan to breastfeed your baby, IF isn't recommended. Just as when you are pregnant, you will be nourishing your baby and for you to do this effectively, you need to make sure that you are eating at appropriate times throughout the day.

- **If you suffer from an eating disorder or you have suffered from such a condition in the past**

If you have anorexia, you are underweight, you have a nutrient deficiency or you suffer from any other kind of eating disorder, it's not recommended to start IF. In fact, any kind of diet that involves food restriction or calorie counting isn't recommended either.

Even if you had suffered from such a condition in the past but you have successfully recovered from it, IF is still not recommended. You might end up feeling stressed because of fasting and this might cause your condition to recur. For either condition, make sure to speak with your doctor about what eating plan you can follow that will benefit you without causing you harm.

- **If you aren't sleeping well or you are experiencing chronic stress**

While IF may benefit you in terms of sleep, if you suffer from poor sleeping habits and you constantly aren't able to get enough sleep each night, changing your eating habits isn't the best idea. Remember that following IF will cause a lot of changes in your body, especially at the beginning. If your poor sleeping habits are already taking a toll on your body, this will make you more susceptible to the potential side effects of IF.

The same thing goes for when you are chronically stressed. If you are always busy or you feel like you are constantly overwhelmed, adding IF to the mix won't benefit you at all. Learn how to manage your stress more effectively first and try to improve your sleeping habits. Then when you start IF, the eating pattern can help improve your life further.

- **If you're completely new to dieting or exercising**

For those who have never tried any kind of diet or who have never exercised in their life, IF might look like the ultimate weight loss solution. While it's true that one of the most significant benefits of IF is weight loss, this eating pattern is quite intense. As I have mentioned, I had already tried other types of diets in the past. So when I tried IF, I wasn't that surprised with the change.

If intermittent fasting is the very first diet you have ever considered, have yourself checked first to make sure that you don't have any existing nutritional deficiencies. Make sure that you start off with a solid nutritional platform first before you start planning.

- **If you suffer from any kind of medical condition**

There are certain medical conditions that will make it difficult for you to start or stick with intermittent fasting. For instance, if you have blood control issues, following IF might exacerbate your condition. Or if you suffer from adrenal issues, IF might push too hard on your adrenal glands which, again, might exacerbate your condition. If you have a history of hypoglycemia, fasting might make you feel lightheaded frequently or constantly irritable.

These are just some examples of conditions that might make IF an unpleasant experience for you. If you suffer from any medical condition, consult with your doctor first. Your doctor is the best person to ask about the new eating pattern you plan to undertake. If your doctor doesn't give you the green light, ask about other diets or eating patterns you can start given your existing condition.

- **Children**

If you plan to follow IF, don't force your children to do the same. Unlike adults, children need nourishment throughout the day to ensure their proper growth and development. Don't force children to fast as this might have adverse side effects on their health.

Just because you don't belong to these groups of people, that doesn't mean that you should start intermittent fasting right away. There are other conditions where you should think twice about starting IF because this eating pattern might not fit into your lifestyle. Seriously consider your choice to start intermittent fasting if:

- **You're married or you have a family**

  Whether you're married without children or you are raising a family with your partner, IF might not fit into your lifestyle. Unless you can cater to their meal schedules while following your own IF plan without getting confused, you may want to rethink your decision.

Imagine if you're the only one on IF in your household. They would share all meals together while you sit on the sidelines because it's your fasting window. This can make you feel bad and it might even make your family feel bad for you. But if you think you can deal with this kind of situation and your family will understand and support your decision, then you may proceed.

- **Your job involves a lot of client interactions or it's performance-oriented**

If you have jobs like these, then you should always be at the top of your game. At the beginning of your IF journey, you may feel weak, lightheaded, or even fatigued. Your energy levels will drop and this might have an effect on your job performance. Of course, these effects will fade away the more you stick with IF so if you think you can deal with it, then you may continue. If not, you may want to think of a different diet or eating plan to follow.

- **You compete in athletics or sports**

competitions

I'm not saying that there aren't any athletes who follow IF because there are. My precaution here is the same as the previous point. The low energy levels you may experience, especially at the beginning, might have an impact on your performance. Consider this before you jump into intermittent fasting.

- **You're a woman**

For this point, you might be raising your eyebrows right now because I am a woman and I follow IF. Unfortunately, when it comes to IF, women should be more cautious because our bodies work differently than men's. For one, fasting might throw your hormones out of balance. As women, we are also more susceptible to the side effects of this eating pattern.

If you suffer from PMS, fasting might worsen your symptoms. Then when you're trying to conceive, you get pregnant or you're breastfeeding, you should stop IF temporarily. Also, women aren't advised to follow the stricter IF methods. But since I am a woman too, I can say that with enough research and awareness, you can safely follow IF. Just make sure that you have considered all the factors carefully and you always put your health first before anything else.

If you don't belong to any of these groups and you know for a fact that you are healthy, then you can go ahead and start IF. Even if you belong to these groups, you may still consider intermittent fasting as long as you communicate openly with your doctor about it. The key here is to know exactly what you are going into. Reading this book is already an excellent first step as you learn all the fundamentals of the diet. With this knowledge, you can start planning your next steps.

Typical Side-Effects of IF

Whether you can freely start intermittent fasting or you should take precautions because you have a condition or you belong to a group of people, the next thing to learn about are the typical side effects you may experience. As with any other dietary change, IF comes with a number of side effects that can be quite unpleasant. Knowing about these will help you prepare for them and know how to deal with them as they come.

Imagine if you had no idea what could happen if you follow IF. Then when you experience any of these side effects, you might panic and decide to quit right away. While most of these side effects will go away over time, if you experience anything severe, it's best to cease your fasting right away. If these side effects come frequently, consider having shorter fasting windows and build up as time goes by. Just give your body time to adapt to your new eating pattern and you'll be fine. Here are the side effects to expect when you start with or continue following intermittent fasting:

- **Hunger and food cravings**

This is the most common side effect of IF and it's also the most obvious. Since you're used to eating at certain times throughout the day, you will definitely feel hungry at some point during your fasting windows. The good news is that we have already discussed some tips and strategies on how you can overcome your urge to eat.

Related to this is a feeling known as "hangry." While this isn't really a word, a lot of people experience this feeling. If you're not familiar with the term, it's a mash-up of the words "hungry" and "angry." Obviously, you would feel hangry when you are so hungry that your emotions (usually anger) get the best of you. When you're hangry, you feel grumpy, grouchy or overall irritability with the world and the people around you. If you're not used to going hungry, you may experience this a lot, especially at the beginning. But just like hunger, "This too shall pass." You can use the strategies I've shared to overcome hunger for this issue as well.

- **Gut or stomach issues**

You may experience issues like bloating, gas, and more when you overeat during your feasting window. This is why I kept reminding you that overeating is never a good idea when it's time for you to eat. Also, try to incorporate more gut-friendly foods into your diet to ensure a healthy gut microbiome. Probiotic foods will help you overcome or even prevent gut issues so try to eat more of these during your feasting windows.

- **Headaches**

This is another common side effect of IF and it is commonly caused by dehydration. As your body adjusts to intermittent fasting, you may experience dull headaches frequently. To ease these headaches or prevent them from happening, make sure to drink a lot of water or calorie-free beverages while fasting.

- **Exacerbation of food sensitivities**

If you have any existing food sensitivities, these could worsen as you start following IF. Some studies have shown that those who have non-celiac gluten sensitivities may develop brain and gut problems while following IF. Other issues that may stem from these food sensitivities are inflammation, weight loss resistance, leaky gut, and more. If you start experiencing such problems, consider taking a break or even changing your IF method until your body adjusts. You can also clean up your diet to prevent any issues related to food sensitivities.

- **Overeating or binge eating**

While these are considered side effects, you can actually control them. As hungry as you are after your fasting window, try not to gorge on food as soon as your feasting window starts. Overeating and binge eating can lead to other issues, so you should try to make a conscious effort to restrain yourself. Again, if you feel like you are ravenous after your fasting window, consider shortening your fasting window until you get used to the concept of not eating. Then you can gradually lengthen your fasting windows over time.

- **Constipation**

Making any kind of change in your diet can cause this side effect. It can even be an indication that you suffer from some sort of medical condition. Drinking more water can help you overcome constipation. This will also go away as soon as your body adjusts to your new eating pattern. If not, have yourself checked.

- **Feeling chilly or cold**

Getting cold toes and fingers while fasting is also a common thing. This is because fasting causes an increase in blood flow to your fat stores. This process is known as "adipose tissue blood flow" and it aids in transporting fat to the muscles where it will be burned for energy. As you fast, you also become more prone to feeling chilly or cold. But you can easily combat this by wearing warm clothes, drinking warm beverages or taking a warm bath.

- **Brain fog or fatigue**

In the beginning, you may experience these side effects. You might find yourself having difficulty concentrating or feeling excessively tired during your fasting hours. This is normal, especially during your adjustment period. After all, you won't be eating anything so your body is still learning how to use your stored fats for energy. To combat this, opt for healthier food choices during your feasting window so these can provide you with energy even while you are fasting.

- **Changes in your mood**

Apart from feeling "hangry," you may experience other unpleasant emotions while fasting. You may even feel these emotions because you feel obligated to follow the schedule you have set for yourself. Like all the other negative side effects, these feelings are normal. Accept them, allow yourself to experience them, and watch as they fade away.

Don't deny these mood changes as doing this might cause them to grow into resentment. If you feel like these mood changes are starting to affect your life, try doing some relaxation or mindfulness techniques. Don't isolate yourself. Instead, connect with other people to distract yourself from the challenges you are experiencing. You can even seek support from a registered nutrition coach, dietitian, or even a psychologist when you are feeling anxious or discouraged. Find ways to make yourself feel better or more positive about IF.

- **Changes in your workout regimen**

Working out while on IF is completely acceptable and safe. In fact, you can use your workouts to distract you from the hunger you feel while fasting. However, don't expect your workout routines to remain the same, especially if you are used to high-intensity exercises. As you are starting out, you may want to tone down your workout regimen so you don't overexert yourself. That way, the other side effects you feel don't worsen, too.

While all of these side effects may fade away over time, you should also know when it's time to quit. Learning how to ease these side effects is one thing, but forcing yourself to endure severe side effects is another. If the side effects don't go away or you're already feeling like something is "off," take a break. If you're starting to feel ill, consult with your doctor. It's all about listening to your body and taking the necessary steps to ensure your overall health and well-being.

Safety Tips for Following IF

Intermittent fasting is one of the most popular and most current health trends all over the world. For the most part, IF is a safe way to improve your health as long as you understand what it is, how to follow it, and how to listen to your body throughout the entire process. It's normal to feel concerned in terms of safety, especially since there are so many different diet trends out there that promise results but end up causing more harm than good.

Perhaps one of the most valuable things I can tell you is that although there have been few IF studies conducted on human beings, most of them have proven the health benefits and positive outcomes of the eating pattern. Combine these results with the many anecdotal reports and you can feel confident enough in the effectiveness and safety of IF. Still, if you really want to make sure that you won't be compromising your health by following IF, consider these safety tips:

- It may be very tempting to jump right into IF so you can enjoy all the benefits, but it's better to ease into the IF method you have chosen. This makes it a more positive and safer experience for you in the long run.
- During your first few fasting windows, allow yourself to eat small amounts of healthy food as needed. Gently push yourself to stick with fasting but don't force it, otherwise, you might experience the adverse side effects of this eating pattern.
- Just because it's called a "feasting window," this doesn't mean that you should literally feast. Unless you plan to follow the warrior fasting method, restrain yourself from eating or indulging too much when it's your eating time.
- Focus on whole foods to improve your health. Although you don't have to restrict or limit any kinds of food when you're not fasting, it's

always better to pair IF with healthier food options.

- Make sure you are well-hydrated all day, every day, whether you're fasting or not.
- Eat sufficient amounts of protein to prevent muscle loss. Just don't go overboard as too much protein can prevent you from entering ketosis.
- Experiment as much as you want until you can find a method that works for you and makes you feel good.
- If you fall ill, stop fasting. Allow yourself to recover before continuing.
- Consider taking supplements to avoid deficiencies. To make sure that you're taking the proper supplements, check with your doctor.

All the other tips and strategies I have shared with you will help you stay safe as you fast intermittently. Just increase your awareness and keep on observing your body for any changes both positive and negative so you can make modifications to your IF plans as needed.

Conclusion: Intermittent Fasting and You

Intermittent fasting isn't just a diet. It's a lifestyle choice that you can consciously make for the purpose of simplifying your life and improving your health. Simple as this eating pattern may be, there's more to it than just cycling between eating and fasting. There are things you must consider if you want to follow IF and there are precautions you must take to ensure your safety.

By now, you already have all the fundamental knowledge you need to decide whether intermittent fasting is the right lifestyle choice for you to make. As I had promised you at the beginning of this book, I've shared with you an objective account of what intermittent fasting is all about. Throughout this book, I have shared information with you based on studies, anecdotal reports, and even some personal experiences from my own intermittent fasting journey. Hopefully, all of this information will help you start and stick with your own IF journey successfully as well.

To help you understand IF better, we started off by defining it and going through its rich and interesting history. Then we went through all of the benefits intermittent fasting has to offer. Just remember that these benefits won't come all at once, nor will you experience them right away. To enjoy the benefits of IF, you must stick with it. As a follower of IF for some time now, I can personally attest to the fact that these benefits are, in fact, real. Even though I haven't experienced all of them, the ones I enjoy now have enriched my life and made me healthier.

Then we discussed the fundamental concepts of intermittent fasting. Knowing these concepts will help you understand IF better and how it works. Next, we went through the most common methods of IF. By learning about these methods, you can determine which one to try depending on your own preferences, lifestyle, and health goals. Then we moved on to a wealth of practical information including tips, pointers, and strategies to help you start and stick with intermittent fasting. Finally, we went through the risks, side effects, precautions, and safety tips. I included this final chapter for you to see the other side of intermittent fasting. I want you to see this eating pattern as a whole, not just the positive side of it. I believe that knowing everything about IF will arm you against all the challenges you may experience while motivating, encouraging, and inspiring you to take your own intermittent fasting journey for the improvement of your life.

I would like to thank you for purchasing and reading this book from start to finish. Hopefully, you gained a lot of insight and learned useful information from the different chapters. My last piece of advice for you is just to stick with it. If you decide to start following IF, go for it! All the benefits are waiting for you, all you have to do is take that all-important first step. Even if you stumble along the way, keep going. Forgive yourself if you make mistakes and keep going. If you believe that this book truly taught you a lot (and I sincerely hope it did), I would love to hear from you. Simply leave a favorable review for me to read along with everyone else out there who is looking or a reliable resource to teach them about intermittent fasting. Good luck on your journey and don't be afraid to inspire others as well.

References:

4 tricks to stick to Intermittent fasting easily. (2019). Retrieved from https://timesofindia.indiatimes.com/life-style/health-fitness/diet/4-tricks-to-stick-to-intermittent-fasting-easily/articleshow/70978326.cms

5 Tips To Make Intermittent Fasting Work For You. (2019). Retrieved from https://evolve-mma.com/blog/5-tips-to-make-intermittent-fasting-work-for-you/

6 religions other than Islam that require fasting. (2016). Retrieved from https://tribune.com.pk/story/1117283/6-religions-islam-require-fasting/

6 Types Of Intermittent Fasting Schedules That Produce Results. (2019). Retrieved from https://evolve-mma.com/blog/6-types-of-intermittent-fasting-schedules-that-produce-results/

Ahmed Atif, L., & Xbiex, T. The concept of fasting in religions. (2009). Retrieved from https://timesofmalta.com/articles/view/the-concept-of-fasting-in-religions.272215

Ahmad, A. Fasting in Religions. (2019). Retrieved from https://www.alislam.org/articles/fasting-in-religions/

Al-Islam, M., Faris, E., Hussein, R., Al-Kurd, R., Al-Fararjeh, M., Bustanji, Y., & Mohammad, M. Impact of Ramadan Intermittent Fasting on Oxidative Stress Measured by Urinary 15- -Isoprostane. (2012). Retrieved from https://www.hindawi.com/journals/jnme/2012/802924/

Ayuda, T. The 4 Most Common Intermittent Side Effects and Health Risks to Know. (2019). Retrieved from https://www.prevention.com/weight-loss/diets/a29758102/intermittent-fasting-side-effects/

Bacharach, E. 12 Fasting Tips That'll Help You Actually Lose Weight (And Not Go Crazy). (2019). Retrieved from https://www.womenshealthmag.com/weight-loss/a29602869/fasting-tips/

Baines, W. 6 Health Benefits of Intermittent Fasting. (2019). Retrieved from https://www.beliefnet.com/wellness/health/6-health-benefits-of-intermittent-fasting.aspx

Bates, A. 3 Ways Intermittent Fasting Can Balance Your Hormones. (2018). Retrieved from https://www.autumnellenutrition.com/post/3-ways-intermittent-fasting-can-balance-your-hormones

Bendix, A. 8 signs your intermittent fasting diet has become unsafe or unhealthy. (2019). Retrieved from https://www.businessinsider.com/signs-intermittent-fasting-unsafe-unhealthy-2019-7#if-youre-feeling-hangry-you-might-want-to-consider-calling-it-quits-8

Berardi, J. Intermittent Fasting: Who's It For? (And, if It's Not for You, What to Do Instead). (2015). Retrieved from https://www.huffpost.com/entry/intermittent-fasting-whos_b_6236712

Berger, M. Intermittent Fasting and Inflammation. (2019). Retrieved from https://www.healthline.com/health-news/fasting-can-help-ease-inflammation-in-the-body

Boyers, L. Intermittent Fasting: What to Know About Fed vs. Fasted States. (2018). Retrieved from https://www.tipsonlifeandlove.com/diet-and-healthy-eating/intermittent-fasting-the-fast-and-the-furious

Bradley, S. Intermittent Fasting Pro And Cons To Consider *Before* You Try It Out. (2019). Retrieved from https://www.womenshealthmag.com/weight-loss/a28905278/intermittent-fasting-pros-and-cons/

Bradley, S. 10 Intermittent Fasting Side Effects That Might Mean It's Not A Great Fit For You. (2019). Retrieved from https://www.womenshealthmag.com/weight-loss/a29657614/intermittent-fasting-side-effects/

Breus, M. What Is Intermittent Fasting, and Will It Help Your Sleep?. (2019). Retrieved from https://www.psychologytoday.com/us/blog/sleep-newzzz/201904/what-is-intermittent-fasting-and-will-it-help-your-sleep

Brueck, H. Skipping a few meals with intermittent fasting may help people avoid cancer, diabetes, and heart disease. (2019). Retrieved from https://www.insider.com/how-intermittent-fasting-prevents-cancer-diabetes-2019-8

Byrne, C. What everyone should know before trying intermittent fasting, according to experts. (2019). Retrieved from https://www.wellandgood.com/good-home/cozy-holiday-gifts-saje/

Cassetty, S. The pros and cons of intermittent fasting. (2018). Retrieved from https://www.nbcnews.com/better/pop-culture/pros-cons-intermittent-fasting-ncna900961

Cerqueira, F., Chausse, B., & Kowaltowski, A. Intermittent Fasting Effects on the Central Nervous System: How Hunger Modulates Brain Function. (2017). Retrieved from https://link.springer.com/referenceworkentry/10.1007%2F978-3-319-40007-5_29-1

Cole, W. Is Intermittent Fasting Bad For Your Hormones? These Are The Pros & Cons. (2019). Retrieved from https://www.mindbodygreen.com/articles/is-intermittent-fasting-bad-for-your-hormones-these-are-the-pros-cons

Collier, R. Intermittent fasting: the science of going without. (2013). Retrieved from https://www.ncbi.nlm.nih.gov/pmc/articles/PMC3680567/

Coulson, C. Stages of Fasting - What Happens When You Fast?. (2019). Retrieved from https://7sigmaphysiques.com/stages-of-fasting-what-happens-when-you-fast/

Cranston, T. Intermittent Fasting, The One Lifestyle To Rule Them All. (2018). Retrieved from https://medium.com/the-ascent/intermittent-fasting-the-one-lifestyle-to-rule-them-all-1cdf3ad1d88d

Diet Review: Intermittent Fasting for Weight Loss. (2019). Retrieved from https://www.hsph.harvard.edu/nutritionsource/healthy-weight/diet-reviews/intermittent-fasting/

Fasted and Fed State. (2017). Retrieved from https://train.fitness/personal-trainer-blogs/fasted-and-fed-state

Fasting to Reverse Fatty Liver Disease: Does it Work?. (2019). Retrieved from http://biomify.com/fasting-fatty-liver-disease/

Feast then famine – how fasting might make our cells more resilient to stress. (2016). Retrieved from https://theconversation.com/feast-then-famine-how-fasting-might-make-our-cells-more-resilient-to-stress-38808

Fletcher, J. Intermittent fasting for weight loss: 5 tips to start. (2019). Retrieved from https://www.medicalnewstoday.com/articles/32488 2.php

Fredericks, K. 7 Proven Benefits of Intermittent Fasting. (2019). Retrieved from https://www.thehealthy.com/weight-loss/intermittent-fasting-benefits/

Fung, J. Fasting - A History. (2019). Retrieved from https://thefastingmethod.com/fasting-a-history-part-i/

Fung, J. The Fed and the Fasted State - The Fasting Method. (2019). Retrieved from https://thefastingmethod.com/fed-fasted-state/

Ganesan, K., Habboush, Y., & Sultan, S. Intermittent Fasting: The Choice for a Healthier Lifestyle. (2018). Retrieved from https://www.ncbi.nlm.nih.gov/pmc/articles/PMC6 128599/

Group, E. The Stages of Fasting: What Happens To Your Body When You Fast?. (2017). Retrieved from https://www.globalhealingcenter.com/natural-health/stages-of-fasting-what-happens-when-you-fast/

Gunnars, K. 6 Popular Ways to Do Intermittent Fasting. (2017). Retrieved from https://www.healthline.com/nutrition/6-ways-to-do-intermittent-fasting

Gunnars, K. Intermittent Fasting 101 — The Ultimate Beginner's Guide. (2018). Retrieved from https://www.healthline.com/nutrition/intermittent-fasting-guide

Gunnars, K. What Is Intermittent Fasting? Explained in Human Terms. (2017). Retrieved from https://www.healthline.com/nutrition/what-is-intermittent-fasting

Gunnars, K. 10 Evidence-Based Health Benefits of Intermittent Fasting. (2016). Retrieved from https://www.healthline.com/nutrition/10-health-benefits-of-intermittent-fasting

Harvie, M., Sims, A., Pegington, M., Spence, K., Mitchell, A., & Vaughan, A. et al. Intermittent energy restriction induces changes in breast gene expression and systemic metabolism. (2016). Retrieved from https://breast-cancer-research.biomedcentral.com/articles/10.1186/s13058-016-0714-4

Hatori, M., Vollmers, C., Zarrinpar, A., DiTacchio, L., Bushong, E., & Gill, S. et al. Time restricted feeding without reducing caloric intake prevents metabolic diseases in mice fed a high fat diet. (2012). Retrieved from https://www.ncbi.nlm.nih.gov/pmc/articles/PMC3491655/

Hicks, C. Why fasting is now back in fashion. (2015). Retrieved from https://www.telegraph.co.uk/lifestyle/11524808/The-history-of-fasting.html

How fasting helps fight fatty liver disease. (2016). Retrieved from https://www.sciencedaily.com/releases/2016/05/160509085347.htm

Intermittent Fasting: 4 Different Types Explained. (2019). Retrieved from https://health.clevelandclinic.org/intermittent-fasting-4-different-types-explained/

Intermittent fasting and its effects on the body and brain. (2019). Retrieved from https://thisnzlife.co.nz/intermittent-fasting-and-its-effects-on-the-body-and-brain/

Intermittent Fasting Implementation FAQ's. (2017). Retrieved from https://www.fasterwaytofatloss.com/blog/2017/3/7/intermittent-fasting-implementation-faqs

Jarreau, P. How to Practice Intermittent Fasting Safely. (2019). Retrieved from https://lifeapps.io/fasting/how-to-practice-intermittent-fasting-safely/

Jarreau, P. The 5 Stages of Intermittent Fasting. (2019). Retrieved from https://lifeapps.io/fasting/the-5-stages-of-intermittent-fasting/

Jordan, S., Tung, N., Casanova-Acebes, M., Chang, C., Cantoni, C., & Zhang, D. et al. Dietary Intake Regulates the Circulating Inflammatory Monocyte Pool. (2019). Retrieved from https://www.cell.com/cell/fulltext/S0092-8674(19)30850-5

Kamb, S. Intermittent Fasting For Beginners: Should You Skip Breakfast?. (2019). Retrieved from https://www.nerdfitness.com/blog/a-beginners-guide-to-intermittent-fasting/

Kandola, A. What are the benefits of intermittent fasting?. (2018). Retrieved from https://www.medicalnewstoday.com/articles/32360 5.php

Kresser, C. Intermittent Fasting: The Science Behind the Trend. (2019). Retrieved from https://chriskresser.com/intermittent-fasting-the-science-behind-the-trend/

Lett, R. 7 Types of Intermittent Fasting, Explained. (2019). Retrieved from https://www.span.health/blog/7-types-of-intermittent-fasting-explained

Lett, R. Guide to Managing Hunger, while Intermittent Fasting. (2019). Retrieved from https://www.span.health/blog/guide-to-hunger-while-intermittent-fasting

Link, R. 8 Health Benefits of Fasting, Backed by Science. (2019). Retrieved from https://www.healthline.com/nutrition/fasting-benefits

Long Fasts: Dangerous or Beneficial?. (2019). Retrieved from https://paleoleap.com/long-fasts/

Longo, V., & Mattson, M. Fasting: Molecular Mechanisms and Clinical Applications. (2015). Retrieved from https://www.ncbi.nlm.nih.gov/pmc/articles/PMC3946160/

Loria, K. The amazing ways intermittent fasting affects your body and brain. (2018). Retrieved from https://www.businessinsider.com/benefits-of-intermittent-fasting-disease-fighting-weight-loss-2018-3#more-research-is-still-needed-on-the-different-forms-of-intermittent-fasting-10

Mattson, M., Longo, V., & Harvie, M. Impact of intermittent fasting on health and disease processes. (2017). Retrieved from https://www.ncbi.nlm.nih.gov/pmc/articles/PMC5411330/

Mattson, M., & Wan, R. Beneficial effects of intermittent fasting and caloric restriction on the cardiovascular and cerebrovascular systems. (2005). Retrieved from https://www.ncbi.nlm.nih.gov/pubmed/15741046

Migala, J. 6 Types of Intermittent Fasting: Which Is Best for You?. (2018). Retrieved from https://www.everydayhealth.com/diet-nutrition/diet/types-intermittent-fasting-which-best-you/

Miller, K. Curious About Intermittent Fasting? This Is Everything You Need To Know To Start The Diet. (2019). Retrieved from https://www.womenshealthmag.com/weight-loss/a28563472/intermittent-fasting-diet/

Mosley, M., & Spencer, M. The Fast Diet: Lose Weight, Stay Healthy, and Live Longer with the Simple Secret of Intermittent Fasting. (2019). Retrieved from https://deanyeong.com/reading-note/the-fast-diet/

Not so fast: Pros and cons of the newest diet trend. (2019). Retrieved from https://www.health.harvard.edu/heart-health/not-so-fast-pros-and-cons-of-the-newest-diet-trend

Nurmasitoh, T., Utami, S., Kusumawardani, E., Najmuddin, A., & Fidianingsih, I. Intermittent fasting decreases oxidative stress parameters in Wistar rats (Rattus norvegicus). (2018). Retrieved from https://univmed.org/ejurnal/index.php/medicina/article/view/462

Oppenheim, S. Is Intermittent Fasting Really The Healthiest Way To Eat? Not For Everyone. (2019). Retrieved (2019). from https://www.forbes.com/sites/serenaoppenheim/2019/01/24/is-intermittent-fasting-really-the-healthiest-way-to-eat-not-for-everyone/#5d8d38a23606

Paddock, C. How fasting boosts exercise's effects on endurance. (2018). Retrieved from https://www.medicalnewstoday.com/articles/321056.php#1

Patterson, R., Laughlin, G., Sears, D., LaCroix, A., Marinac, C., & Gallo, L. et al. INTERMITTENT FASTING AND HUMAN METABOLIC HEALTH. (2015). Retrieved from https://www.ncbi.nlm.nih.gov/pmc/articles/PMC4516560/

Pattillo, A. Is Intermittent Fasting "Natural"? History Experts React to the Controversy. (2019). Retrieved from https://www.inverse.com/article/57835-intermittent-fasting-evolution

Pavilonis, V. Science unclear on intermittent fasting. (2019). Retrieved from https://yaledailynews.com/blog/2019/09/26/science-unclear-on-intermittent-fasting/

Pedre, V. Intermittent Fasting Can Be Dangerous For Some People. Here's Exactly What You Need To Know. (2019). Retrieved from https://www.mindbodygreen.com/0-29932/intermittent-fasting-can-be-dangerous-for-some-people-heres-exactly-what-you-need-to-know.html

Pera, V. Intermittent Fasting: Does It Work and Is It Safe?. (2019). Retrieved from https://www.lifespan.org/lifespan-living/intermittent-fasting-does-it-work-and-it-safe

Redman, L., & Ravussin, E. Caloric Restriction in Humans: Impact on Physiological, Psychological, and Behavioral Outcomes. (2011). Retrieved from https://www.ncbi.nlm.nih.gov/pmc/articles/PMC3014770/

Self Compassion: your secret weapon to ditch diet
    culture.   (2019).   Retrieved   from
    https://eatwithawareness.com/self-compassion-
    your-secret-weapon-to-ditch-diet-culture/

Sboros, M. Simplicity of intermittent fasting is making it
    a   popular   diet.   (2019).   Retrieved   from
    https://www.businesslive.co.za/bd/life/2019-10-
    28-marika-sboros-simplicity-of-intermittent-fasting-
    is-making-it-a-popular-diet/

Simplicity: Why Intermittent Fasting is so Damn
    Effective.   (2011).   Retrieved   from
    https://cavemantoday.wordpress.com/2011/06/09
    /why-intermittent-fasting-is-so-effective/

SINKUS, T. Intermittent Fasting Daily Plan. (2019).
    Retrieved   from
    https://21dayhero.com/intermittent-fasting-daily-
    plan/

Sugar, J. 9 Common Side Effects of Intermittent
    Fasting (and How to Deal). (2018). Retrieved from
    https://www.yahoo.com/lifestyle/9-common-side-
    effects-intermittent-013529487.html

Sugar, J. If You Want to Try Intermittent Fasting to Lose Weight, Do These 7 Things. (2018). Retrieved from https://www.popsugar.com/fitness/How-Start-Intermittent-Fasting-44867509

Talens, D. How to Free Yourself from Food Cravings with Intermittent Fasting. (2015). Retrieved from https://vitals.lifehacker.com/how-to-free-yourself-from-food-cravings-with-intermitte-1702108722

Tello, M. Intermittent fasting: Surprising update. (2018). Retrieved from https://www.health.harvard.edu/blog/intermittent-fasting-surprising-update-2018062914156

The 7 Different Types of Intermittent Fasting, Explained. (2018). Retrieved from https://perfectketo.com/types-intermittent-fasting/

The Benefits of Short Term Fasting. (2019). Retrieved from https://chosenfoods.com/blogs/central/the-benefits-of-short-term-fasting

The surprising benefits of intermittent fasting. (2019). Retrieved from https://www.cbhs.com.au/health-well-being-blog/blog-article/2019/04/11/the-surprising-benefits-of-intermittent-fasting

Tomic, M. How to Deal with Hunger During Intermittent Fasting: Leangains. (2019). Retrieved from https://shockingfit.com/hunger-intermittent-fasting-leangains/

Virgin, J. Why Intermittent Fasting Is The Best Thing To Ever Happen To Your Metabolism. (2019). Retrieved from https://www.mindbodygreen.com/articles/why-intermittent-fasting-is-the-best-thing-to-ever-happen-to-your-metabolism

Wei, M., Brandhorst, S., Shelehchi, M., Mirzaei, H., Cheng, C., & Budniak, J. et al. Fasting-mimicking diet and markers/risk factors for aging, diabetes, cancer, and cardiovascular disease. (2017). Retrieved from https://www.ncbi.nlm.nih.gov/pubmed/28202779

West, H. How to Fast Safely: 10 Helpful Tips. (2019). Retrieved from https://www.healthline.com/nutrition/how-to-fast

Why is Fasting Back in Fashion? The Spiritual History Behind Today's Diet Trend. (2018). Retrieved from https://medium.com/@ifcj/why-is-fasting-back-in-fashion-the-spiritual-history-behind-todays-diet-trend-4273b3fd4ab

Why the Intermittent Fasting 16/8 Method Might Be Right For You. (2019). Retrieved from https://perfectketo.com/how-often-should-you-intermittent-fast/

Williams, C. What Is The Obesity Code Diet—And Can It Help You Lose Weight?. (2018). Retrieved from https://www.cookinglight.com/eating-smart/nutrition-101/the-obesity-code-review

Williamson, A. Evidence Backed Benefits of Intermittent Fasting. (2019). Retrieved from https://medium.com/infinite-mindspace/top-five-evidence-backed-benefits-of-intermittent-fasting-f827fdb7ee54

Zauner, C., Schneeweiss, B., Kranz, A., Madl, C., Ratheiser, K., & Kramer, L. et al. Resting energy expenditure in short-term starvation is increased as a result of an increase in serum norepinephrine. (2000). Retrieved from https://www.ncbi.nlm.nih.gov/pubmed/10837292